D0511679

praise for Jorge and *8 minutes in the morning*

'The number one excuse for not working out is "Time!". Well, now you have no excuse because Jorge Cruise has the solu   r both time and body, 8 Minutes in the Morning!'

— **Tamilee Webb**, MA, star of *Buns of Steel* video series

'How great is this p   nme?!? Jorge's is an incredibly easy plan that produces real weight loss and fitness improvemen   ss than 10 minutes a day, right at home – without gyms, personal trainers, or special foods and su   nents. If you want to get fit, firm, and feel better about yourself – even if you've never been s   ssful before – you owe it to yourself to give this programme a try!'

Catherine Cassidy, editor-in-chief of *Prevention* magazine

'Hooray for Jorge! A   , a weight-loss expert who explodes misconceptions about fat and introduces how the "right" fat   make you fit. Hold on for a slimmer and healthier you.'

Jade Beutler, author of *Understanding Fats and Oils*

'If you can't take 8 m   es out of a 24-hour day to take care of the most important person on this Earth, you are just plain lazy. Jorge will get you up and started.'

Jack LaLanne, host of the first nationally syndicated US TV exercise show and 'The Godfather of Physical Fitness'

'Jorge wants to get you super-healthy, not just super-lean.'

Lisa Klugman, editor-in-chief of *Fit* magazine

0042360404

8 minutes
in the
morning®

Stockton Borough
8|03
Public Libraries

00 4 236040

Part three: The Programme

Part four: Resources

you've got the power

By Anthony Robbins, author of *Awaken the Giant Within*

Congratulations on your commitment to improving the quality of your life! I truly believe that physical health and vitality are the basis for an outstanding life, and I guarantee that when your body is in optimum condition, you will enjoy amazing energy, allowing you to grow, contribute to others, and lead a fulfilling and passionate life. With such energy, your possibilities are limitless. Not only will you feel outstanding physically but also you will have a mental clarity that will enable you to focus on taking control of your future and making your dreams a reality.

Remember: your body is not your enemy! Many people, in their desire to be high achievers, create immense amounts of stress for themselves. Unfortunately, food becomes the vehicle by which they alleviate that stress, and the result is poor health and often a feeling of discouragement or even desperation.

We all know that we should change our habits to improve

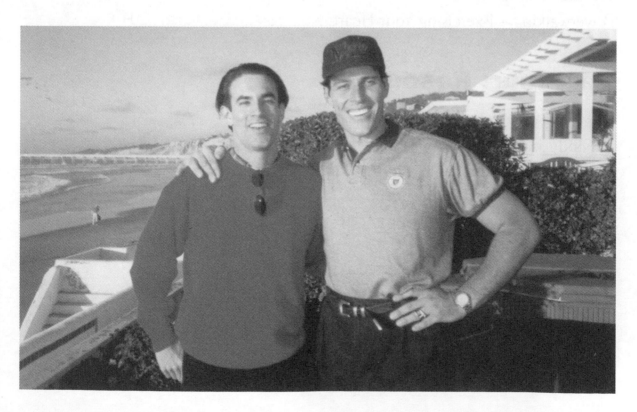

'Working with someone who understands your frustrations and can encourage you in overcoming the challenges along the way will keep you on track and even accelerate the pace at which you achieve your desired results.'

our lifestyles. What happens is that we make the decision to begin a new health programme, but then something else comes up and we don't have time. We quit. The reason we encounter such challenges is because this decision is a 'should', not a 'must'. And as I tell people all the time, we are constantly 'shoulding' all over ourselves. Unless our decision becomes a part of who we are – our identity – the changes we make will be only temporary.

Once health becomes a must, there is something else I recommend to help people stay focused: coaching. Working with someone who understands your frustrations and can encourage you in overcoming the challenges along the way will keep you on track and even accelerate the pace at which you achieve your desired results.

Jorge Cruise's *8 Minutes in the Morning* can be that coach.

Jorge (left) with bestselling author Anthony Robbins

Jorge Cruise decided long ago to end his unhealthy habits and restore vitality and passion to his life. He knows the struggles involved in getting and staying healthy; therefore, he understands the importance of support. *8 Minutes in the Morning* sets you up to win. Jorge is with you each step of the way, but by the end of the 4-week programme, the only person you will need is you.

8 Minutes in the Morning effectively supports your decision to make health and fitness your top priorities. You will learn how to achieve optimum health and how to attack the process with organization, consistency and emotion. Time spent exercising is minimized, while your energy is maximized, creating the momentum necessary to propel you towards the body you desire and deserve.

Remember, it is in our moments of decision that our destiny is shaped. I commend and respect you for taking action towards giving yourself the gift of extraordinary health and vitality.

introduction to a new life

by ann-marie carpenter, jorge client

I did nothing for more than 10 years. I felt tired and depressed and weighed 4 st 4 lb (27 kg) more than I should. And it definitely was not extra muscle. After I found out that I was a grandmother at the age of 57, I decided to make sure that I was going to live long enough to not only watch my granddaughter grow up but also have a quality relationship with her. I had to lose the weight and get fit, and I had to start immediately.

I know how you may be feeling right now. I had no energy or time to start a 'programme'. I was tired all the time, and I felt more depressed whenever I saw my reflection in the mirror. It had been 15 years since I exercised regularly, followed a healthy diet or really even thought about weight loss. Back then, I had only 2 st 12 lb (18 kg) to lose. I changed my habits and lost the weight, but within 3 months, I gained it all back, plus 1 st 6 lb (9 kg). That didn't help my spirits.

Still, I went online to look for a weight-loss plan that I thought I could stick with, and I came across a site that promised me that I could 'lose weight and get fit and healthy in only 8 Minutes in the Morning'. I figured I would try that. After all, 8 minutes was less time than I spent flipping through channels during TV commercials. The programme certainly was a lot cheaper and simpler than all of the potions, pills and concoctions I'd read about, too. So I ordered Jorge Cruise's programme.

Jorge's programme made exercising and eating easier. I got fitter, and I lost weight. I was consistently losing – every 2 weeks, I recorded a 5 lb (2.25 kg) loss! I had lots of energy, and I was feeling great about myself.

Just 5 months later, I had lost 3½ st (22 kg). I was down to a size 14 and had not felt deprived for a minute. This programme has helped me change my outlook on life. Even after I reached my goal weight, I continued with 8 Minutes in the Morning. Now I am a new me!

I have maintained my weight and my energy level, and Jorge Cruise's programme has become a part of my life. The best part about 8 Minutes in the Morning is that anyone can do it. If a grandma at the age of 57 can do it, then anyone can do it! There is nothing magical about my success; *you* can do the same with 8 *Minutes in the Morning*. If you make the commitment to take the time for yourself, you can join me in a new life of being fit and healthy, and I guarantee that you will be happier than you have been in a long time.

Thank you, Jorge, for my new life.

'If a grandma at the age of 57 can do it, then anyone can do it!'

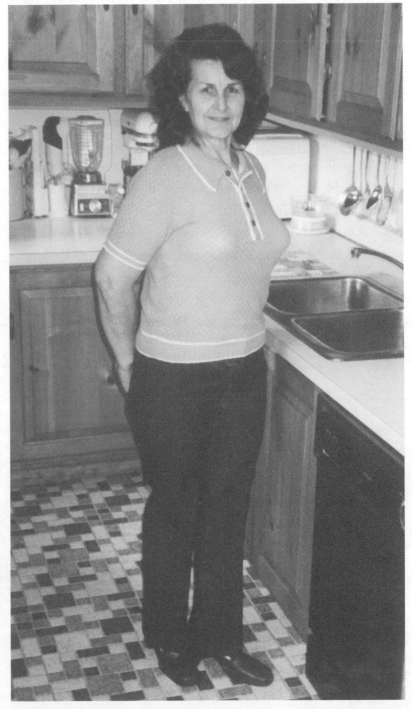

before

after
I lost 2 to 2½ pounds (1 kg) each week – 5 pounds (2.25 kg) every 2 weeks! You can achieve the same results!

get ready to start

Welcome to 8 Minutes in the Morning, the number one weight-loss programme for people who don't have time. I want to congratulate you and thank you for selecting me to be your coach.

How is your life about to change? Why will you get hooked on this programme for life? My philosophy is simple: losing weight does not take a lot of time and is not hard when you use the most effective and proven techniques.

This programme is the result of my coaching more than 3 million cyberspace clients.

I created it based on their feedback and success stories specifically for people who are time-deprived but want rapid results. If you don't want to spend hours in the gym but do want to look as if you do, my programme is for you. If you don't want to wait forever to see results, my programme is for you.

Here is my promise to you:

follow my programme, and you will see amazing results with just 8 Minutes in the Morning. Everything you need is within these pages. Get ready for an adventure that will change your life and body forever. I look forward to hearing your success story soon.

Your coach,

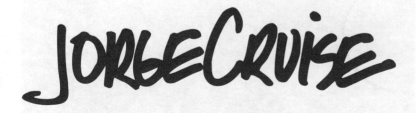

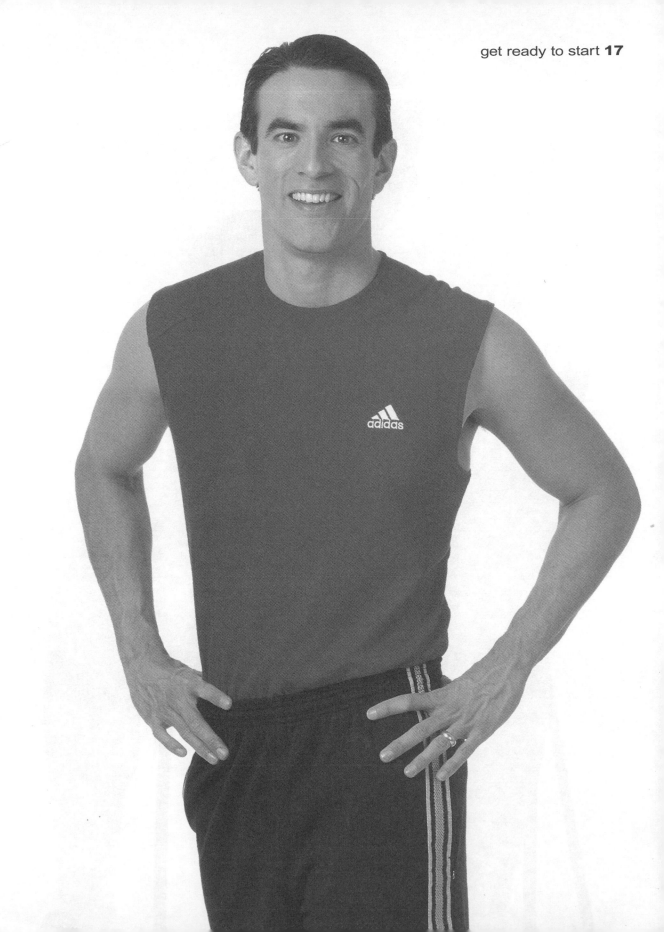

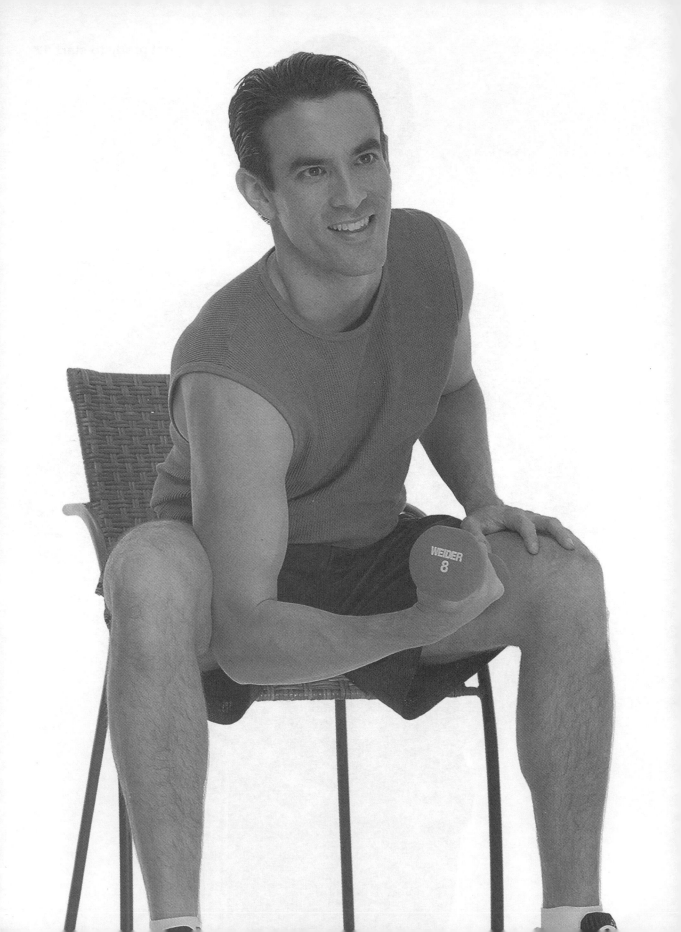

1
Jorge and You

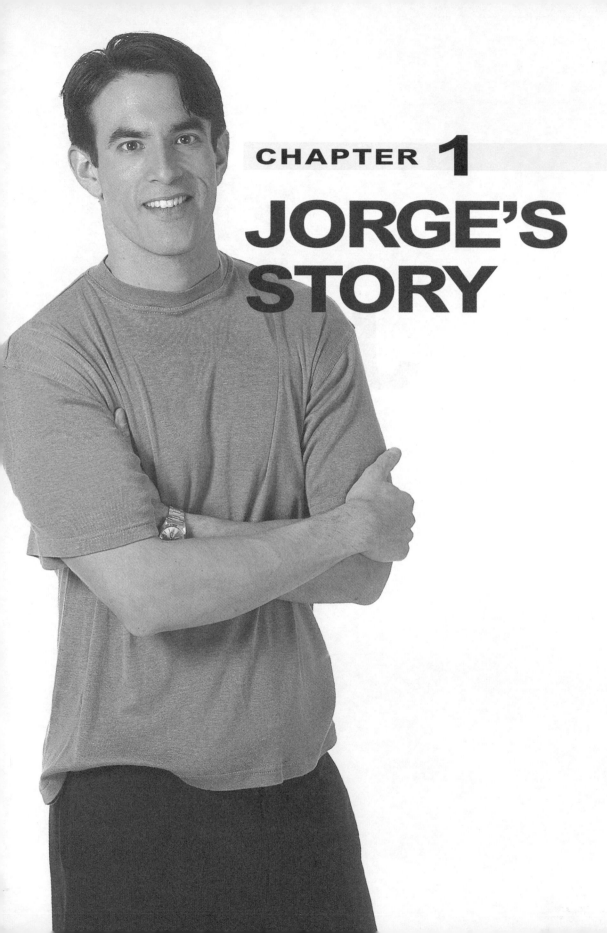

CHAPTER 1
JORGE'S STORY

the birth of 8 minutes in the morning

There isn't a day that goes by that I don't remember what my life was like before I decided to change my body and make weight loss a priority. I am very grateful when I think of how far I've come. Believe me, it's amazing how great your life can be once you feel good inside and out.

'I know what it is like to be embarrassed by extra weight.'

This is why I do what I do. I know that no matter what riches you may have, if you are unfit and unhealthy, you have nothing. This is why I have dedicated myself to empowering others with the best and most effective exercise programme: my 8 Minutes in the Morning.

You may think that I have always been Mr Fitness, that I have always been addicted to being in great shape, but neither of these things is true. I know what it's like to be embarrassed by extra weight – and worse. I know because I've been there. My dad has been there. So have my sister and my grandfather. We were all fat and unhealthy. And now we're not.

the 'king' of poor health

I grew up in Southern California with a mother from Mexico City and a father from Pennsylvania. Both sides of my family loved rich foods: cheese, milk, cream, anything fried, sausages and red meat – all served up in huge portions.

Basically, my family had two key beliefs that were wrong. First, they believed that how much you ate equalled how much you were loved. And because my mom and grandma loved me so much, they both fed me a lot. My mom would feed me one meal and then my grandma would almost always offer me another. I showed my love by eating those huge portions. I probably ate enough food for three kids. At home, I consumed enormous quesadillas, bologna sandwiches and nachos. When we ate out, it was usually at fast-food restaurants, where all my meals were oversized.

If I didn't eat everything on my plate, my mom or grandma would take it very personally. I can't explain why love somehow becomes so intertwined with food. Maybe for my grandmother it dated back to her childhood years when she was poor and sometimes didn't have enough food. Maybe she wanted to make sure that her grandchildren never had to go through the same kind of childhood.

I got so chubby that my mom used to call me *el rey*, which in Spanish means 'the king', and before long, I looked more like King Arthur's table: round.

My family also believed that exercise was hard and time-consuming. My mom and dad were very busy, both working 10-hour days. We *never* exercised. And I don't think anyone in my family ever thought anything was wrong with the way I looked. To my grandmother, the fat on my bones was a sign of health, not a sign of weakness.

Consequently, by the time I was 15, I was a physical disaster. I had low energy, daily headaches and severe asthma. No one – certainly not my family – ever suspected that my health challenges were caused by my lifestyle.

As I gained weight, I became less active. At school, when it was time to pick teams to play kickball or softball or football, I was always the last kid chosen. I don't think I ever flunked gym class, but I sure didn't do well. I know what it's like to be so unhealthy and unfit that you feel like a reject – a nothing – especially when the kids let you know that they think you're no good. I remember those Presidential Physical Fitness Tests where the gym teacher would make us to do as many situps, pullups and pushups as we could. I never could do one. Not one.

I went along in this state until I almost died. Yes, you read it right. I had been suffering from a bad stomach-ache for several weeks. I tried drinking lots of water and herbal teas, but it didn't help. I couldn't eat and quickly started losing weight. A trip to casualty when the pain worsened revealed that a piece of meat had become lodged in my appendix, causing it to burst.

From then on, I tried to change the way I ate, but I didn't know how. The whole concept of healthy eating and exercising was completely foreign to me.

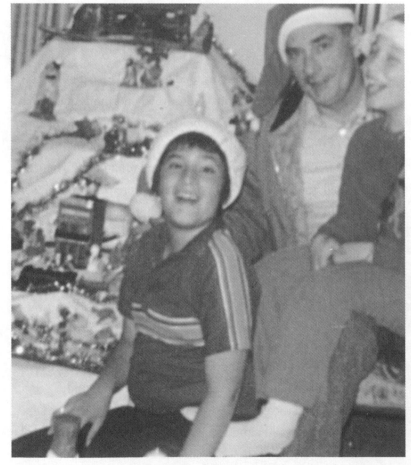

Here I am on the road to an unhealthy life. If I had not changed my eating patterns, I would have easily weighed more than 14 st (90 kg).

hitting too close to home

At 18, something happened that made me change my eating and exercise habits for good. My dad was diagnosed with prostate cancer, and the doctors gave him a death sentence. They told him that with no medical intervention, he had 1 year to live. They predicted that if he had his prostate surgically removed and went through a chemotherapy and radiation treatment regime, he might last 5 to 6 years. My dad knew that surgical removal of his prostate would probably make him incontinent as well as destroy his sex life, so he decided to forgo medical intervention.

That was 1989, and he's still alive and healthy. Instead of undergoing surgery, chemotherapy and radiation, my dad dramatically changed his lifestyle. He enrolled in an alternative health centre in San Diego where people go to learn about lifestyle changes that promote cleansing, rejuvenation and healing.

I was so shaken up about his cancer that I went with him. I figured that the cancer was probably genetic, and if I didn't take action, I could well be facing the same disease. At the centre, Dad and I learned all about nutrition. We learned which foods contain fibre and which ones don't, about the value of whole grains over processed foods, about fruits and vegetables, about healthy fats, and about herbs such as wheat grass. We discovered that dairy products can cause allergic reactions in some people.

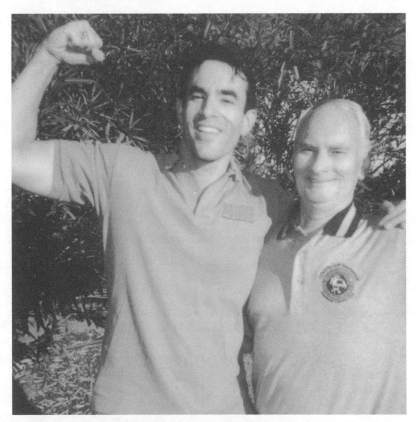

Today my dad is 2 st (13 kg) lighter and healthier than ever.

adopting a new lifestyle

I stopped eating so much dairy and red meat, switched from processed foods to whole grains and veggies, started drinking more water and eating soya products, and stopped eating oversized hot dogs and hamburgers. One day, I realized that my headaches were gone, and so was my asthma. I was feeling healthy and energetic. I started to exercise, and I enrolled in the University of California, San Diego, to study exercise science and nutrition.

Dad and I weren't the only ones in my family to change our ways. Everyone was turning over a new leaf. Like me, my sister Marta had also been an overweight child.

She continued to gain weight as she grew older, especially during college. Her weight left her depressed, and her lack of confidence was apparent to everyone who met her. But when she changed her eating habits and started exercising, the weight just fell off. Every time I see her, she's looking more fit and toned.

a second chance

In Pennsylvania, my paternal grandparents were dealing with their own problems. They had always followed an unhealthy diet, and when my grandfather retired, they ate even more. They were both significantly overweight, but they didn't think anything of it until my grandmother suffered her first stroke. While she was recovering in the hospital, my grandfather went in for a check-up. The doctor told him to get his affairs in order. At 5 ft 7 in (1.70 m) and 15 st (95 kg), his blood pressure was 180/110, and the doctor assumed that in a short time, he'd be next to have a stroke.

That shook my grandparents up. They knew about my dad's success and decided that adopting his new lifestyle might help them as well. Unfortunately, it was a little too late for my grandmother. They had decided to move to San Diego, but shortly after they arrived, she suffered a second stroke and died.

The new lifestyle showed dramatic results for Grandpa, however. Within months, he lost more than 3½ st (22 kg) and lowered his blood pressure to 139/89. He had been given a second chance. At the age of 95, he feels great, and he and my dad look more like brothers.

'I now know in my heart that my mission in life is to help people get healthy and stay healthy.'

a message of love from me to you

At college, I was busy studying exercise science and swiftly moving from one extreme to the other. I would hit the gym every day, lifting weights that worked the same muscle groups. I knew that exercise was good, but I didn't know that too much

could be bad. I ended up constantly tearing my muscles and not giving them enough time to recover between sessions. Even though I was eating well and working out, I felt tired all the time. But as my exercise science knowledge grew, I

realized that there can be too much of a good thing.

I learned that lesson again a few years later, when my mom – the one person in our family who had lived a fit lifestyle – developed hip problems. In Mexico City, she had been a

8 minute marvel Marta lost 3 st (19 kg)!

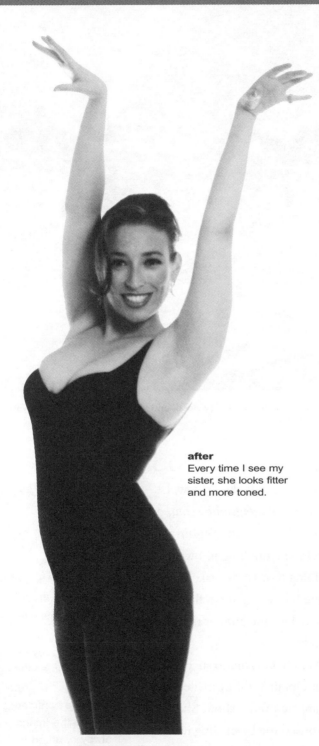

Meet Jorge's sister, Marta, who joined her brother and father on the path to health.

'I now feel incredible and have attracted the man of my dreams!'

after
Every time I see my sister, she looks fitter and more toned.

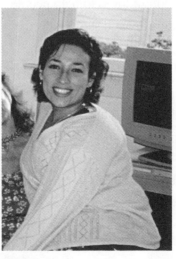

before

professional dancer, and in her early sixties, she started feeling more and more hip pain. She was diagnosed with osteoarthritis. Essentially, the high-impact dancing she had done most of her life had damaged the cartilage that cushioned her hip joints.

Doctors gave her high dosages of painkillers for a year before operating. The painkillers ate away at her kidneys and other body organs. Two years after her hip replacement, my mother died in my arms.

Her death reinforced even more my calling to study exercise science and nutrition. I now know in my heart that my mission in life is to help people get healthy and stay healthy. I want to create a revolution, so I have dedicated my life to empowering others with the best and most effective weight-loss information.

This is why I became certified as a fitness trainer by the Cooper Institute for Aerobics Research, the American College of Sports Medicine (ACSM) and the American Council on Exercise (ACE).

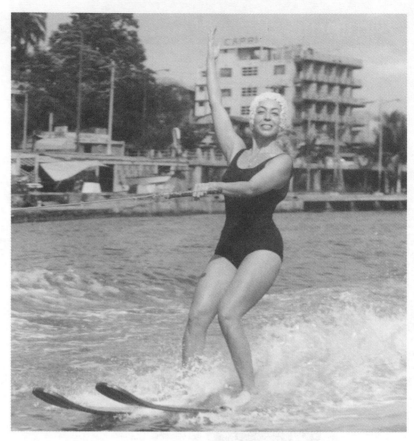

My mom and I were very close, and her passing reinforced my life's mission to empower others.

about the programme

After getting the know-how, I created *www.jorgecruise.com*, my weight-loss website. Within weeks of launching it, I was helping thousands make the same lifestyle changes that had worked for me and for my family.

My site became so successful that Oprah Winfrey invited me to appear on her show. She surprised me by inviting two people to appear on the show

'8 minutes' edge

By training with me in the morning, you will:

- Lose 2 lb (1 kg) of fat per week on average!
- Feel your muscles getting firm!
- See your body develop curves – in all the right places!
- Gain the confidence to go out and do the things you've always wanted to do!

who had transformed their lives with the help of the information on my site.

After that show, my online business and career took off. Soon, millions visited the site regularly, trying the techniques I suggested and giving me feedback about what worked for them and what didn't. People told me that with their work and families, they just didn't have time for long trips to the gym, hour-long aerobics sessions or complicated eating plans. They wanted simplicity.

I made a deal with some of these clients. I would train them personally as long as they allowed me to experiment on them. They would have to try exercises, eating plans and a motivational programme that I would give them. In exchange, they had to let me know what worked and what did not. The result was 8 Minutes in the Morning.

My website also started to address the needs of busy people. I wrote articles and did webcasts about time-efficient exercise programmes and then sought feedback from my clients. Together, we shaped the programme into an

overwhelming success.

Will 8 Minutes in the Morning do the same for you? Absolutely. You will see guaranteed rapid weight loss when you follow my programme.

It does not take a lot of time to get lean as long as you consistently use the most effective exercises. 8 Minutes in the Morning is all you need.

'I have dedicated my life to empowering others with the best and most effective weight-loss information.'

how it works

Follow my 8 Minutes in the Morning programme and you will see amazing weight-loss results in just 28 days. But it doesn't stop there. I will also give you the tools you need to stay lean for the rest of your life. You will be working on three things every day:

Your emotional fitness. Before your 8 Minutes in the Morning routine, I will help you build your own inner motivation with my daily Wake-Up Talk. It will give you the Emotional Advantage you need to move beyond self-sabotaging thinking and motivate yourself to love your new fit lifestyle.

Your physical fitness. My proven 'two superquick moves' are the centre of the programme. They take only 8 minutes a day, but the results are tremendous. Each day, I will give you two new strength-training moves specifically designed to help you speed up your metabolism, get firm, and burn fat as efficiently as possible.

Your eating habits. My Eat Fat to Get Fit nutrition programme is simple to follow and will never leave you feeling deprived. You won't have to count calories or cut out your favourite foods.

Finally, 8 Minutes in the Morning connects you to a community of your peers. I invite you to visit my website at *www.jorgecruise.com* to get more advice from me and to chat with the millions of others who, like you, are well on their way to achieving new health and happiness.

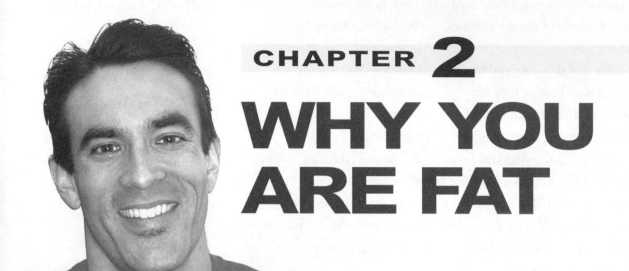

CHAPTER 2
WHY YOU ARE FAT

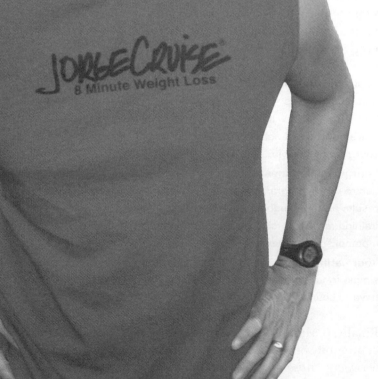

we have all been misled

Since the early 1980s, when the term aerobics came into vogue, hundreds of exercise programmes have been launched to help people get lean. Perhaps you've tried step aerobics, slide aerobics, kickbox aerobics, or even just walking, jogging or running.

'In the UK 51 per cent of the population is overweight.'

Despite all the publicity these different aerobics programmes have received over the years, many people are still fat – and they're getting fatter at an alarming rate. Currently, more than 60 per cent of the total US population is overweight. And nearly one-quarter are clinically obese. And it's not just in America. According to the Worldwatch Institute, the figure is 54 per cent in Russia; in the United Kingdom, 51 per cent; and in Germany, 50 per cent. What is even sadder is that juvenile obesity is also rising rapidly. In many western countries, the incidence of obesity among children has more than doubled over the last 30 years.

According to former Surgeon General C Everett Koop and the Center for Disease Control and Prevention (CDC), more than 300,000 Americans die each year from obesity-related illnesses – second only to 400,000 for tobacco.

This means each day, over 800 Americans die from problems related to obesity. That is the equivalent of 6 airliners with 133 people on board fatally crashing daily. This means that just

the consequences of obesity

Obesity increases the risk of the following:

- Premature death
- High blood pressure
- Diabetes and insulin resistance
- Gallbladder disease
- Kidney disease
- Liver disease
- Heart disease
- Many types of cancer
- Arthritis
- Orthopaedic disorders
- Fatal respiratory disease
- Stroke
- Gout

- Asthma
- Back pain
- Shortness of breath
- Sleep apnoea and snoring
- Reproductive disorders (menstrual problems, female infertility, miscarriage, gestational diabetes)
- Unhealthy cholesterol levels
- Impaired immune function
- Depression
- Chronic pain
- Impaired mobility

within this next hour, 34 people will die. Think about it . . . about every 5 minutes, three people die due to problems related to obesity.

The average woman gains 9 lb (4 kg) between her 30th and 39th birthdays; the average man gains 4 lb (1.8 kg). It is this type of extra weight that puts you at an increased risk of disease. (See 'The Consequences of Obesity', page 29).

It is estimated by the World Health Organization that up to one-third of cancers of the colon, breast, prostate, kidney and digestive tract are due to obesity and lack of exercise.

The bottom line is that the fatter you are, the higher your chance of dying prematurely.

where aerobics falls short

Although aerobic exercise is essential for strengthening your heart and lungs (the cardiovascular system), it is not the most effective way to get lean. You burn roughly 100 calories for every mile that you walk or run. To lose 1 lb (0.5 kg), you would have to walk or run 35 miles (56 km).

And aerobic exercise is not so practical if you are overweight. It can be too uncomfortable. Even walking can be difficult because your joints may start to ache, and you can get out of breath very quickly. Before coming to me, almost all of my clients had given up exercising because the aerobic approach was too difficult for them. Plus, if you focus on aerobics, your body

shape will stay the same, even if you burn enough body fat. If you are currently shaped like a pear, you will look like a smaller pear. You'll lose weight first where you don't want to – your breasts – and last where you do want to – your thighs. Your body will still feel flabby and, worse, your skin will probably sag.

But the exercises in my 8 Minutes in the Morning programme will help you burn fat and improve your body shape. You will tone your shoulders so that your waist looks narrower. Your arms will be smaller as well as firmer. Your abdominal muscles will be not only leaner but stronger, and they'll provide better support for your torso.

'It is estimated by the World Health Organization that up to one-third of cancers of the colon, breast, prostate, kidney and digestive tract are due to obesity and lack of exercise. The bottom line is that the fatter you are, the higher your chance of dying prematurely.'

I'm not saying that you shouldn't do *any* aerobic exercise. Beyond my 8 Minutes, I recommend that you incorporate some aerobics into your lifestyle because you need to keep your heart and lungs strong. Plus, it reduces stress. For tips on beginning the most convenient type of aerobic exercise, see the chapter on powerwalking on page 204.

why starvation dieting doesn't work

You have been told that dieting is the key to weight loss, that weight loss is simple – just don't eat. And research shows that you can fairly easily lose unwanted weight by starving yourself. The problem is that up to 50 per cent of that weight comes from muscle tissue loss, not from fat loss. This sets you up for disaster.

Here's what happens. When you don't eat enough, your thyroid gland (located in your neck) tries to protect you from starvation. It secretes less thyroxine, a hormone that helps regulate your metabolism. The less thyroxine you have, the slower your metabolism and the fewer calories you burn. If you continue this stringent diet for a long period of time, your body will eventually start to consume itself. You may think that this is wonderful because, after all, you do want to slim down. But half of that weight loss will have come from lean muscle tissue.

Your muscle tissue is your body's metabolic furnace. Every pound of muscle burns roughly 50 calories a day. Every pound of muscle you lose on a diet means that your metabolism slows by 50 calories a day. As your metabolism slows down, you'll have to eat less and less food to compensate. Eventually, weight loss becomes extremely difficult and you hit that all-too-familiar plateau. Few people can continue to eat so few calories for any length of time. As soon as you start eating normally again, your body will regain the weight you just lost. And because nearly all of that regained weight goes straight to your fat cells, your metabolism will stay sluggish. This is why many people who lose weight end up gaining back more than they lost.

For many people, muscle is already in perilously short supply. What you don't use, you lose. And a convenience-driven lifestyle of escalators, remote controls and jumping into the car every time you go shopping takes a huge toll on your muscle mass over time. As you lose muscle, your metabolism grows more sluggish. This is why people tend to grow fatter as they age. Even if you don't gain weight, you may still get fatter because heavier, more compact muscle tissue is replaced by lighter, more expansive fat tissue. You weigh the same when you get on the scales, but your trousers no longer fit.

Fortunately, there is a better way. If starving yourself and huffing and puffing through hours of aerobics didn't give you the belly, backside and thighs – or the health benefits – of your dreams, then it's time to try the most efficient and quickest way to get lean: my special combination of superquick strength-training moves and the Eat Fat to Get Fit eating system.

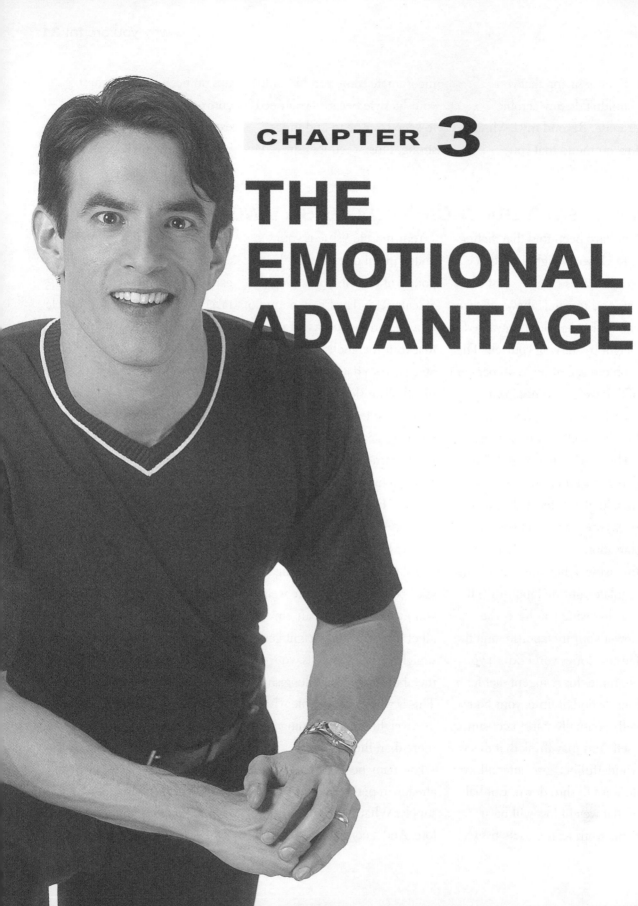

CHAPTER 3

THE EMOTIONAL ADVANTAGE

your firm foundation

To lose weight with 8 Minutes in the Morning, you must first get what I call an Emotional Advantage. In my work with millions of clients online, I've learned that emotional and physical health go hand in hand. Most people can't lose weight and keep it off until they also lose their negative emotions. Once they get fit emotionally, it's like magic. Everything else becomes just a walk in the park.

'In my work with clients, I've learned that emotional and physical health go hand in hand.'

So no matter what genetic pack of cards you have been dealt, an Emotional Advantage will help to ensure you have a *successful and fun weight-loss journey.* With it, you will not only lose weight and build strength but also you will feel your confidence soar.

How can I guarantee that you will really lose the weight this time, and keep it off? Well, millions of my online clients have been exactly where you are, and now they are fit and firm.

special cases

While almost everyone can benefit from an exercise programme like 8 Minutes in the Morning, there are instances when caution is called for.

- If you are pregnant, please consult your doctor before undertaking a rigorous fitness regime. Pregnancy brings on a whole host of changes in your body, increasing your need for a number of nutrients and making some types of exercises – especially those that involve lying on your back – dangerous for you and your baby.
- If your children are younger than 18 years old, their bodies are going through many changes, so my programme should be adapted to their individual needs and their exact stage of development. Please discuss with your doctor the idea of including your children in your workout.
- If you have diabetes, it is safe to use my programme. The food boxes on the Eating Card (see page 74) follow the same exchanges, or caloric values, as the American Diabetes Association. Discuss the programme with your doctor or a registered dietitian, but in most cases, you can gain the benefits of the 8 Minutes in the Morning programme.

8 minute marvel Amber lost 1½ st (9.6 kg)!

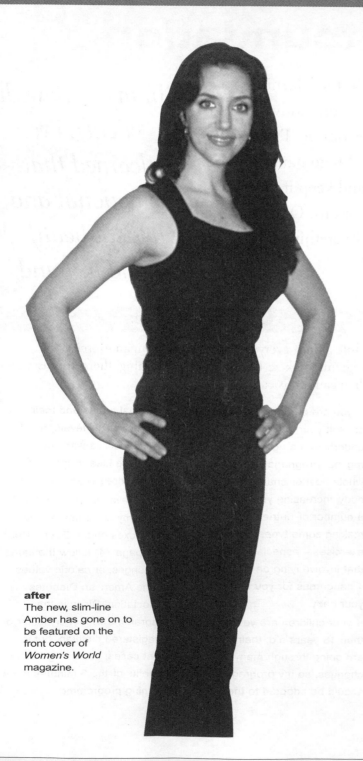

This programme helped me change my old self-sabotaging habits to ones that support my growth. The mental exercises have helped me look into my heart and soul to find what I need in this life.

'It was the easiest weight I ever lost. I love that it only takes me 8 minutes in the morning to do my routine.'

after
The new, slim-line Amber has gone on to be featured on the front cover of *Women's World* magazine.

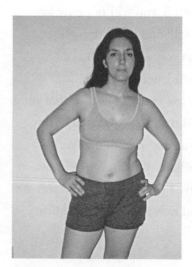

before

full, but unfulfilled

I'd like to tell you a story about Amber Dunlap, a client who was one of my first Emotional Advantage test cases. She started dieting when she was a teenager, gaining and losing the same 10 to 15 lbs (4 to 7 kg) in an effort to become thin enough to be a model. 'I was miserable. I was constantly depressed and struggling to keep the pounds off,' she told me.

As the years went by, her depression magnified and her weight increased. 'I decided that if I were going to get big, I might as well eat all of the foods that I had denied myself for so long.' And she did.

'Then one day, I caught a glimpse of myself in a glass door. I saw more than an out-of-shape woman. I saw an empty soul. I felt so unfulfilled, and I had no idea how to change it.'

After spending 4 weeks building her Emotional Advantage, she told me, 'Emotionally, I feel so in control. This programme helped me change my old self-sabotaging habits to ones that support my growth. The mental exercises have helped me look into my heart and soul to find

what I need in this life. I have faith in myself and my ability to change what I can for my success.'

getting fit from the inside out

Think of all the exercise and weight-loss programmes that you have started – and then stopped. At the beginning, you felt so confident, so excited, so sure that this time you were going to see results. This time you were not going to fall off the weight-loss wagon.

How long did that feeling last? Two weeks? Three weeks? Or just 2 days?

For any exercise or weight-loss programme to work, you must stay with it. I'm going to teach you how to make the positive feelings last much longer – for the rest of your life.

You will see dramatic weight loss in just 4 weeks, and you will get hooked on doing the 8 Minutes in the Morning programme. I guarantee that your motivational drive will grow stronger every day with a simple system to keep you focused so that you stay

'How you feel controls your behaviour.'

consistently inspired to take action.

You will become more fit on the outside by firming up and losing fat, but you'll also become fit on the inside. And when you get fit from the inside out, you'll tap storehouses of motivation and confidence that you didn't know you had.

Think about it. If you perceive exercise as a chore, odds are that you won't exercise consistently. If you think of eating well as punishment, you probably won't eat well consistently. How you *feel* controls your behaviour and directly affects your physical fitness. When something makes you feel extraordinary, you do it effortlessly. If you feel unfocused, unmotivated and tired, you don't. Will you snack on an apple or a piece of cheesecake? Will you wake up early to exercise or sleep in? Go for a vigorous walk or drop in front of the TV after work? The key to automatically choosing the healthier option is knowing how to manage your emotions. That's where the Emotional Advantage comes in.

wake-up talk

Each day, before you start your 8 Minutes in the Morning strength-training moves, you'll spend a few minutes getting focused and emotionally inspired with a Wake-Up Talk. These will infuse your strength training with the Emotional Advantage and help you feel consistently motivated to take action. Through these talks, you will:

- Identify your weight-loss goals – IDENTIFY!
- Discover new incentives for shedding those pounds – DISCOVER!
- Transform yourself from a negative thinker into a positive thinker – TRANSFORM!
- Create a secret energy source by changing the way you breathe
- Use the power of visualization to change your actions
- Free up time that you didn't know you had
- Boost your mood in just 1 second
- Unveil your self-confidence

These short talks will change your outlook on life. Until now, you've been thinking like a fat person. Your Wake-Up Talks will teach you how to think like a thin person. These talks take just a few moments each day to do, but by the end of the initial month-long programme, you'll feel happy, confident, driven, committed and focused. The Emotional Advantage will help you not only stick with the 8 Minutes in the Morning programme but it will actually help you look forward to it!

the write stuff

In addition to your morning Wake-Up Talk, you'll find Today's Journal – another daily feature of the 8 Minutes in the Morning programme. Use this space to record your progress, your breakthroughs and what you are grateful for in your life. This book is meant to be interactive and cannot be finalized without your input. Writing your goals and thoughts will personalize your programme. It's a simple yet effective process. One of the most powerful ways you learn is from yourself, and keeping a journal will teach you more

Today's Journal
Today was great. I got up early enough to do the programme and actually eat breakfast at home instead of at work. I want to try to do this more often…it starts my day much more calmly. Jan asked me to run a few errands with her at lunch, so I suggested we walk instead of drive. We got our aerobic activity in at the same time! I did eat chocolate today, but only 2 of those miniature-size bars, so I feel good about that. All in all, it was a great day… if I keep it up, I'll be in that new outfit at next weekend's get-together. I'm looking forward to what my relatives and friends will think of the new me!

about you. So keep a pen handy and add your notes to each day's journal. When you add the information that is uniquely yours, this book automatically becomes the most important book in your library.

When I started using the daily journal as part of my programme, there was an overwhelming response from my clients. It became a permanent positive feature of 8 Minutes in the Morning. Perhaps Oprah Winfrey said it best: 'Keeping a journal will absolutely change your life in ways you've never imagined.'

Use your journal to write about:

- How you feel
- Your energy level
- What you did well today, such as a positive thought you had or a positive action ('I had some candy-coated chocolates today and stopped at just three!')
- The foods you ate or any new recipes you tried
- How you are progressing in the programme (include the details)
- The positive benefits of your continuing weight loss ('Bob told me I looked great today.')

Use this journal as a log of your personal journey. Whether you write a paragraph or fill up a page, get into the habit of listening to your inner thoughts and writing about how you feel. After the 4-week programme, I'm going to ask you to read through your journal entries so that you can see how far you've come.

getting started

To jump-start the building of your inner emotional strength, do the following three simple things right now.

Take Your 'Before' Photo

Most people tell me that they hate having their 'before' photos taken. What they mean is that they hate having *any* photos of themselves taken. Yet my clients often e-mail me and thank me for having encouraged them to do it. Having that photo taken is such a basic action, yet it signals a change deep inside you. As soon as that photo is developed, it becomes the 'before' photo, starting you on your journey to your 'after' photo.

It's such a simple distinction, but such a strong symbol. You would not believe how many of my clients tell me how their attitudes about weight loss changed almost instantly just because they took that 'before' picture. It's a symbol of your commitment. It's a symbol of your new beginning.

tips from the photo pros

It is in your best interest to take a great 'before' photo. The better the quality of the photo, the more accurately you'll be able to assess your progress.

1 Have your photo fill the frame as much as possible without cutting off body parts.
2 Use a quality camera and film.
3 Use a background that is medium to light in colour.
4 Take the picture in good light, either in the early morning or late evening.
5 Keep the camera angle the same on your 'before' and 'after' photos.
6 Use the same pose as you will for your 'after' photo.
7 Keep your original photo and negatives in a safe location.

Your photo is a powerful reminder of your progress, and that's motivating! Clients say that on their worst days, they would look at their 'before' photos and feel instantly inspired.

Finally, that photo will hold you accountable to the programme. Your 'before' photo is one of the most important tools you will ever use. It will remind you of your amazing progress for years to come. You will remain grateful and inspired for life. Look at it periodically and tell yourself, 'That's the old me.' Your 'new me' is finally emerging!

Decide What You Want

Clarity is power. You need to have focus to achieve your goals, according to author Tony Robbins, my friend and mentor. He taught me that to get what you want in life, you must first know what you *specifically* want. Too often, he says, if you ask someone what she wants, you'll hear instead about what she doesn't want.

To illustrate his point, he shared this story. Tony was invited to learn how to drive a racing car. He was surprised to learn that most injuries come from not successfully coming out of spins.

His instructor told him that the key to coming out of a spin is to focus on where you want to go. Instead, most people focus on what they fear – the wall – and so that's where they go.

Even though Tony had been told this, the first time he went into a spin, his eyes went straight to the wall. His instructor had to grab his head and move it to where the car needed to go. Sure enough, as he focused in that direction, he couldn't help but turn the steering wheel accordingly.

Weight loss is a lot like driving that racing car. In order to get results, you must focus on where you want to go. Saying what you don't want – 'I don't want to be fat' – is not going to get you there. That's like looking at the wall. To get what you want, you must focus on what you want. Yet, saying, 'I want to lose weight' is not as effective as saying, 'I want to lose 10 pounds this month'. The second gives you clarity and focus. It also gives you a deadline.

But don't choose your goal randomly. It must be realistic. To estimate your ideal weight, look at 'Finding Your Ideal Weight' on page 40. Once you know your

goal weight and the approximate date you will achieve it, keep yourself motivated by doing the following.

Weigh yourself every week. Don't be afraid to get on the scales. It is important for you to track your weight-loss progress. Weigh in on Sundays, ideally first thing in the morning before you eat. Your weight may fluctuate due to water retention and the amount of food in your stomach, so don't panic if every once in a while it seems as though you haven't made much progress.

To see your true progress, use the 'Success Chart' on page 41. Use it to plot your weight loss each week. Once you connect the dots, you'll see that, overall, your weight is dropping.

Use a tape measure. It's helpful for you to track the inches you are losing. This will keep you motivated and on track. Remember that muscle is more compact than fat, and you will be increasing your lean muscle tissue as you burn away fat. You will be replacing fat with muscle, so you will see a significant difference in inches even if you don't see a dramatic loss in weight. Your clothes will feel looser as you become fitter.

TRACKING YOUR SUCCESS

Before you go any further, take the time to assess where you are now so you can compare it with where you'll be. This is another really good thing to do that all my clients love. You will, too.

Tape your 'before' photo here. (Double-sided tape works best.)

Today's date: _____

Tape your 'after' photo here.

Today's date: _____

Body Measurements

Right arm:_____   Left arm:_____

Bust/Chest:_____   Neck:_____

Waist:_____   Hips:_____

Right thigh:_____   Left thigh:_____

Weight:_____

Body Measurements

Right arm:_____   Left arm:_____

Bust/Chest:_____   Neck:_____

Waist:_____   Hips:_____

Right thigh:_____   Left thigh:_____

Weight:_____

FINDING YOUR IDEAL WEIGHT

Find your age and height on the chart. You know yourself better than anyone else does, so select a number that is realistic for you. Subtract that number from your current weight. That's your weight-loss goal. Write the number on this line: _____

Work out a target date for achieving your weight-loss goal. On the 8 Minutes in the Morning programme, you can expect to lose fat at a sensible and safe rate of 1½ to 2 lb (up to 1 kg) a week, which is what doctors recommend. Some people lose 3 to 4 lb (up to 2 kg) in a week. So to lose 56 lb (4 st or 25 kg)

of fat, it will probably take you about 25 weeks. That means sticking to the programme for only 5 to 6 months. The great news is that you will start to see results in just 28 days.

Divide the amount of weight you want to lose by 2 (the average number of pounds most people lose each week). The

result is about the number of weeks it should take you to reach your goal weight. Or, if you are working in kilos, the number will equal the number of weeks it will take. Write this number and the date by which you will achieve this new weight on the line below. (Get your calendar out if you need to and find the date.)

_____ pounds (kilos)   by _____ (date)

Height	Weight (lb/kg)		Height	Weight (lb/kg)	
	19–34yr	35+yr		19–34yr	35+yr
5'0" (1.52 m)	6 st 13 lb–9 st 2 lb (44–58 kg)	7 st 10 lb–9 st 12 lb (49–63 kg)	**5'8"** (1.72 m)	8 st 13 lb–11 st 10 lb (57–75 kg)	9 st 12 lb–12 st 10 lb (63–81 kg)
5'1" (1.54 m)	7 st 3 lb–9 st 6 lb (46–60 kg)	7 st 13 lb–10 st 3 lb (50–65 kg)	**5'9"** (1.75 m)	9 st 3 lb–12 st 1 lb (59–77 kg)	10 st 2 lb–13 st 1 lb (65–83 kg)
5'2" (1.57 m)	7 st 6 lb–9 st 11 lb (47–62 kg)	8 st 3 lb–10 st 8 lb (52–67 kg)	**5'10"** (1.77 m)	9 st 6 lb–12 st 6 lb (60–79 kg)	10 st 6 lb–13 st 6 lb (66–85 kg)
5'3" (1.60 m)	7 st 9 lb–10 st 1 lb (49–64 kg)	8 st 7 lb–10 st 12 lb (54–69 kg)	**5'11"** (1.80 m)	9 st 10 lb–12 st 11 lb (62–81 kg)	10 st 11 lb–13 st 12 lb (69–88 kg)
5'4" (1.62 m)	7 st 13 lb–10 st 6 lb (50–66 kg)	8 st 10 lb–11 st 13 lb (55–71 kg)	**6'0"** (1.83 m)	10 st–13 st 2 lb (64–84 kg)	11 st 1 lb–14 st 3 lb (70–90 kg)
5'5" (1.65 m)	8 st 2 lb–10 st 10 lb (52–68 kg)	9 st–11 st 8 lb (57–74 kg)	**6'1"** (1.85 m)	10 st 4 lb–13 st 7 lb (65–86 kg)	11 st 5 lb–14 st 9 lb (72–93 kg)
5'6" (1.67 m)	8 st 6 lb–11 st 1 lb (54–70 kg)	9 st 4 lb–11 st 13 lb (59–76 kg)	**6'2"** (1.88 m)	10 st 8 lb–13 st 13 lb (67–89 kg)	11 st 10 lb–15st (75–95 kg)
5'7" (1.70 m)	8 st 9 lb–11 st 6 lb (55–73 kg)	9 st 8 lb–12 st 4 lb (61–78 kg)	**6'3"** (1.91 m)	10 st 12 lb–14st 4lb (69–91 kg)	12st–15st 6lb (76–98 kg)

Source: US Department of Health and Human Services, *Dietary Guideline for Americans*

SUCCESS CHART

Starting at zero, chart your weight loss on the graph. The horizontal line lists weeks and the vertical line keeps a running total of pounds/kilos lost or gained.

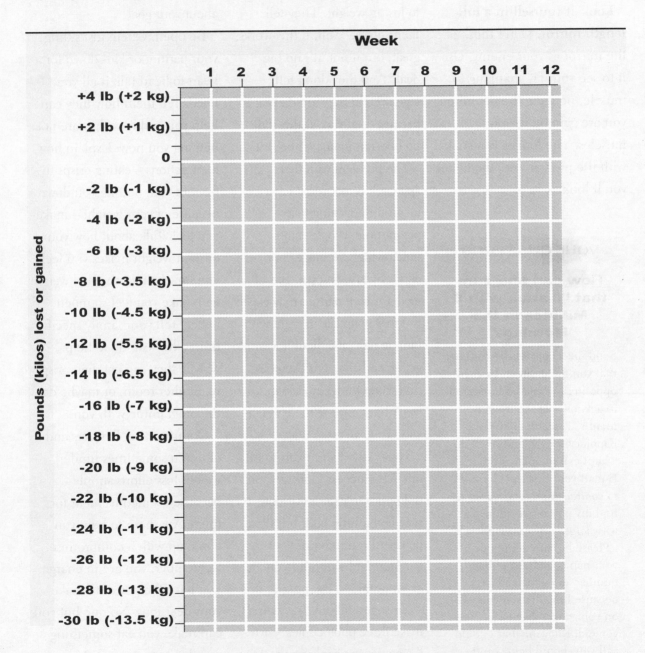

Measure just below your belly button and any other areas you want to monitor, such as your thighs, arms or neck.

Look at yourself in a full-length mirror. Don't think of the mirror as your enemy. Use it to see your fat changing to muscle, noticing the definition you are gaining in your muscles. The longer you stick with the programme, the better you'll look.

your questions

How can I be sure that I'll stick with 8 Minutes in the Morning?

Send me a copy of the contract that you filled out and signed opposite. I would be honoured to acknowledge your commitment to a healthier and happier lifestyle, and I will do what I can to hold you to it. E-mail your Success Contract to *contract@jorgecruise.com* or find my post office address at *www.jorgecruise.com/mail*.

Please be sure to include your name, address, phone number and e-mail address because I might even call you on your target date to see how you did. Knowing that I could call you should help you stay on track!

Commit Yourself To Success

Too many people commit themselves only half-heartedly to losing weight. They tell themselves, 'Well, if this works, great, but if not, it's no big deal.' And they don't tell anyone that they are dieting because that way, if they fail, no one has to know about it.

The problem with that approach is that you'll have a tough time sticking to a programme. People may unknowingly sabotage your efforts by bringing you gifts of food. Or your partner may expect you to stay up late at night with him, making it difficult for you to get up early for your exercises. And when things are rough, you won't have anyone there to tell you, 'You can't stop now.'

That's why I want you to fill out 'My Success Contract' on the opposite page right now. It may feel a little odd, but it's a powerful reminder of your decision and will hold you accountable to the programme.

Once you fill out the contract, make three photocopies. Give the copies to people you feel you can trust and share your plans with them. Explain to them how you intend to lose the weight and tell them how they can help. Here are a couple of tips for talking to friends and family about your goal.

Be open. Often, just sitting your partner or kids down for a heart-to-heart talk is all you need. Tell them how they can help you and how they are not helping you now. Explain how their actions – eating crisps in front of you, putting you down because of your weight – make you feel. Talk about how your current weight makes you feel and how being your goal weight will make you feel so much better. Tell your family specific things they can do to help. Maybe they can eat their crisps in another room, or maybe do the programme with you.

Compromise. Partners and children sometimes hinder weight-loss efforts simply because it's inconvenient for them. Ask them to help you come up with a compromise. Remember, you are in charge. You have the power to make your decisions. No one but you can make you eat something you don't want to eat. No one but you can force you to skip your 8 Minutes in the Morning.

my success
contract

Filling out this contract is one of the important first steps in the 8 Minutes in the Morning programme. Make three copies and give them to trusted friends who will support and motivate you in your journey to success.

Name:_____

Today's date:_____

I am going to lose this many pounds/kilos: _____

By this date:_____

_____
Signature

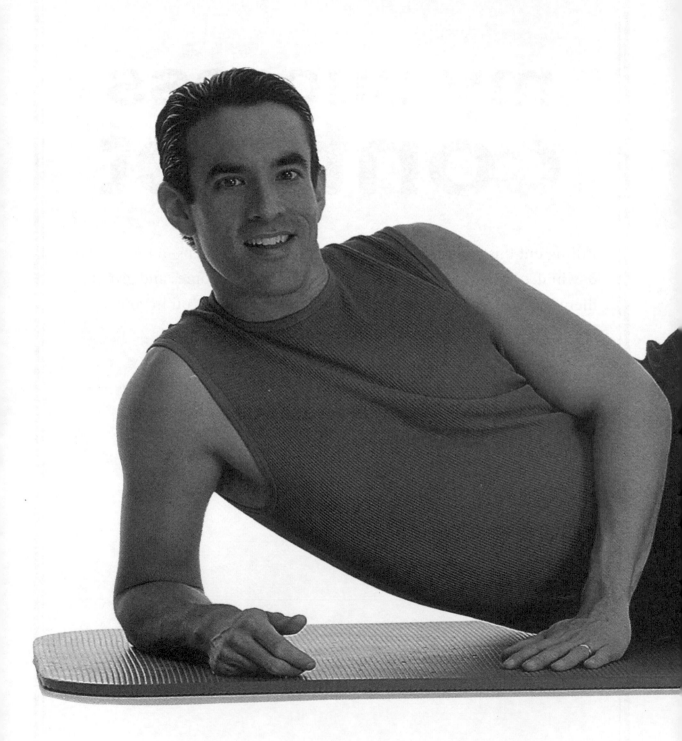

2
How It Works

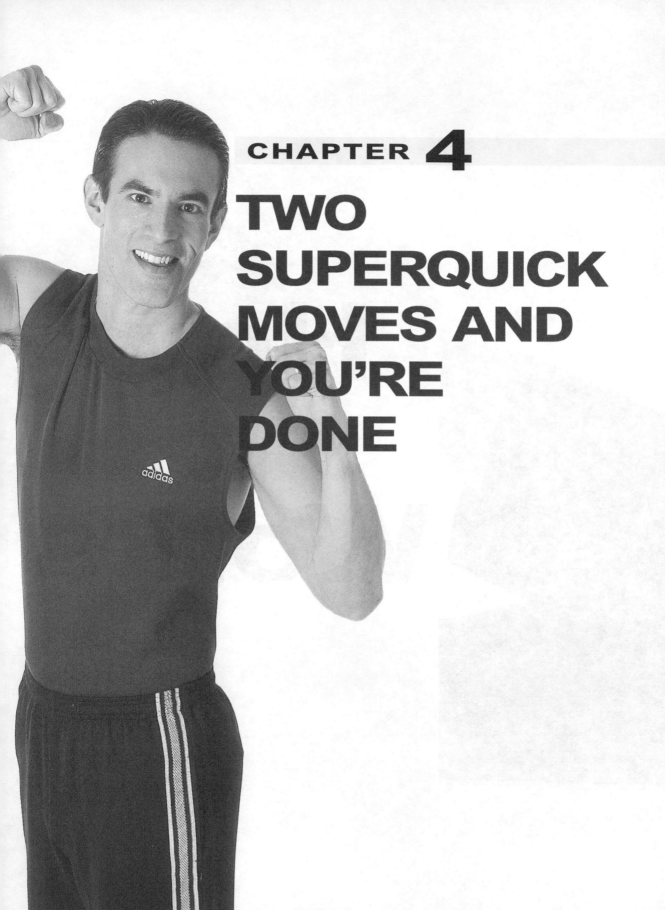

CHAPTER 4

TWO SUPERQUICK MOVES AND YOU'RE DONE

getting lean fast

It's no wonder that people think exercising is too hard and takes too much time. During various attempts to lose weight and firm up, they have forced themselves to sweat it out for half an hour or more and, worst of all, saw few results. It does not take a lot of time to get lean if you consistently use the most effective exercises. And just a couple of the right efficient fat-burning moves will give you unbelievable results. This is the core of my 8 Minutes in the Morning programme.

'The most effective exercise programme for losing weight is a morning strength-training session.'

The most effective exercise programme for losing weight is a morning strength-training session. This is absolutely critical for you to know! Your true problem is not excess fat; that's just the symptom. The underlying problem is a lack of lean muscle tissue. Why? The single most important factor that determines how much fat you burn throughout the day is the amount of lean muscle tissue in your body. The more lean muscle tissue you have, the more efficiently your body burns fat. (See chapter 5, starting on page 52, to understand the fat-burning power of the morning.)

Rev Up Your Fat Burner
Imagine that you are a Volkswagen Beetle but your mechanic has upgraded your engine to a more powerful one from a Porsche. Would this

your '8 minutes' edge

Strength training is the smart way to lose weight because it's also good for your overall health. New research shows that strength training:

- Increases bone density, helping to prevent osteoporosis
- Improves your balance, preventing falls and injuries
- Lowers your blood pressure, cholesterol levels, and risk of stroke, diabetes, cancer and arthritis
- Boosts your metabolism to burn fat 24 hours a day
- Raises energy levels for a more active lifestyle
- Promotes a better mood and better sleep patterns with the release of endorphins
- Brings an end to yo-yo weight loss and gain

stronger engine consume more fuel? Yes. The same is true when you strength train. You create more muscle (a stronger engine) and burn more fat (your fuel).

In addition to creating stronger muscles, strength training also creates a stronger metabolism. That's because lean muscle tissue is very 'active' and requires more calories to survive. Lean muscle tissue is a 'calorie eater' and will help you get and keep a lean body. The more lean muscle tissue you have, the more body fat you will burn!

Imagine you added 5 lb (2.25 kg) of lean muscle tissue over the next few months. (Pound for pound, muscle takes up a lot less space than fat.) You would then be burning an additional 250 calories a day without changing your diet. That means that you would be burning over 25 lb (11 kg) of fat each year you maintain the muscle. And remember that on my programme, you will be building up lean muscle tissue and following my Eat Fat to Get Fit nutritional programme. When you put these two components together, you will see guaranteed results – an average of a 2 lb (1 kg) weight loss each week. Normally, when you lose weight, you lose 75 per cent of it as fat and 25 per cent of it as muscle. But when you do strength training, you lose nearly all fat and no muscle. Lean tissue derives 75 to 95 per cent of its energy from body fat, so for every new pound of muscle you build, you incinerate about 50 additional calories per day. The more lean tissue you have, the more body fat you will shed – even at night, while you sleep. So instead of burning just 60 calories of fat per hour while sitting in a chair at work, you now burn 120 calories of fat per hour doing the same thing.

Feel Younger and Stronger

Besides looking better, you're going to feel better, too. You'll feel younger because strength training turns back the ageing clock. According to a study of postmenopausal women, the body becomes 15 to 20 years more youthful after just 1 year of strength training. Strength training also encourages you to exercise more throughout the day.

And once your muscles become stronger – usually by week 2 or 3 – you will find yourself suddenly doing things you never thought possible. You'll opt to take a walk in the evening instead of sitting in front of the television, you'll want to take the stairs at work, and you'll get up from behind that desk to take quick walking breaks throughout your work day. You'll ignore escalators and moving walkways in favour of your own two feet. All of this will accelerate your results.

And remember what I said about aerobic exercise being too challenging when you're overweight? That's not true for strength training. There will be

your questions

Will the strength-training exercises in your 8 Minutes in the Morning programme make me look like a weightlifter?

Ladies, don't worry about bulking up. Women don't produce as much of the growth-producing hormone testosterone as men do – men produce up to 30 times more. Female bodybuilders follow a very different training programme and achieve 'he-man' looks only with steroid use. I promise that your muscles will become firmer, sexier and shapelier – not bulkier.

no uncomfortable huffing and puffing with my programme. Apart from a few sets of dumbbells, you will need no special clothing or equipment, either. Even if you have never succeeded in losing weight with aerobics or other exercise programmes, I guarantee that you'll do great with 8 Minutes in the Morning – and that 8 Minutes in the Morning will make you feel great!

how strength training works

Once you start my 28-day programme, you'll work two different groups of muscles each day. Sunday is your day off.

Each day of the programme brings you two new exercises. And this is one of the most unique aspects of the 8 Minutes in the Morning programme. The way I've combined these exercises allows you to constantly challenge your muscles in new ways. Each day, you'll break down muscle tissue, which is a good thing. It's how your body grows. After your workout, your body goes to work to repair that lean tissue, making you stronger. The next time you lift the same weight, it won't feel so heavy. This muscle-repair stage is called the afterburn. Your metabolism will stay revved up for hours after your 8 Minutes in the Morning: 7 to 12 per cent higher for 15 or more hours, which amounts to 600-plus incinerated calories. After you do aerobic exercise, your metabolism returns to normal within an hour, burning only 15 to 50 additional calories.

your questions

While I have the weights in my hands, can I add some repetitions to increase the effects of my 8 Minutes in the Morning workouts?

The strength-training exercises included in the 8 Minutes in the Morning programme are designed to work in sync with the nutritional intake values that are indicated with the Eating Card System (see page 74). A better fitness move for you is to challenge your body with aerobic activities, starting with my powerwalking programme on page 204.

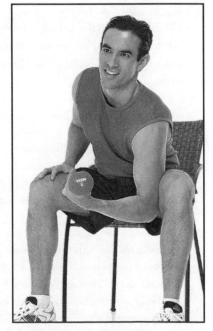

When you're deciding which weights to buy, take the biceps curl test (see over).

daily exercise

monday
chest and back

tuesday
shoulders and abdominals

wednesday
triceps and biceps (arms)

thursday
hamstrings and quadriceps (legs)

friday
calves and buttocks

saturday
inner and outer thighs

choose your weights

To do your 8 Minutes in the Morning exercises, all you'll need are some dumbbells, a chair and a towel or mat. I strongly recommend that you purchase three pairs of dumbbells: a light pair, a medium pair and a heavy pair. This will ensure that you work both your smaller and larger muscles effectively.

To work out which weights to buy, take the biceps curl test.

your questions

What Makes 8 Minutes of Strength Training So Smart?

The type of strength training in my programme is perfect for busy people. Here are just a few of the unique reasons why 8 Minutes in the Morning is the most effective way to lose weight.

• My programme encourages you to strength train in the morning. When you strength train in the morning, as opposed to later in the day, you will immediately elevate your metabolism for the whole day. After your 8 Minutes in the Morning session, your body will be working hard to start building your lean tissue, and that will seriously boost your metabolism. And that's only one of many benefits of morning exercise.

• Other strength-training programmes have you spending 40 minutes or more in the gym, but my programme contains a special series of moves that take only 8 minutes a day. I specifically designed and tested this workout based on the feedback of millions of my online clients. They told me that they didn't have time for the trip to the gym and that they wanted to work out at home without buying fancy equipment.

• My proven moves are the most efficient combination of strength-training moves around. I tested them on my online clients. They work. By consistently challenging different muscle groups every day, you'll give your metabolism the biggest boost possible.

• I have combined my strength-training moves with two other bonus components that will further maximize your weight loss. I call the first one the Emotional Advantage. It's the motivational component of 8 Minutes in the Morning, and it will keep you on track. The second is my breakthrough eating programme called Eat Fat to Get Fit. For guaranteed success on your 8 Minutes in the Morning programme, you must use all three aspects of the programme at the same time.

1 Select a weight that you think you can curl 12 times without stopping.

2 With a dumbbell in each hand, repeatedly curl the weight.

3 If you can curl more than 12 times, the weight is too light. If you can't reach 12 repetitions, the weight is too heavy. If you can do 12 repetitions but not 13, you've found the right middle-range weight.

4 To select your lighter weights, subtract 2 to 3 lb (1 to 1.5 kg) from your middle-range weight. For example, if you selected 8 lb (3.5 kg) as your mid-range dumbbell, you would most likely select a 5- or 6-lb (2- to 2.5-kg) dumbbell as your lighter one.

5 To select your heavier dumbbell, add 2 to 3 lb (1 to 1.5 kg) to your mid-range dumbbell. If your mid-range weight were 8 lb (3.5 kg), you should most likely select a 10-lb (4.5- to 5-kg) dumbbell.

You can find dumbbells weighing up to 20 lb (9 kg) in department stores. For heavier weights, you will need to go to a sports shop. Second-hand weights are OK.

8 Minute Marvel the Raymond family lost 33 lb (15 kg)!

After we found Jorge's programme, we decided to make it a family project. This is something that we can all benefit from and support each other in. We get up and do the exercises together, which takes less than 15 minutes a day!

'We're getting active as a family, which has enriched our lives and brought us closer.'

So far, Sam has lost 1 st 2 lb (7.2 kg), I have lost 10 lb (4.5 kg) and Nicolas has lost 7 lb (3.2 kg). We have more strength and energy, and even sleep better.

Carrie Raymond

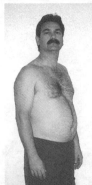

Sam before

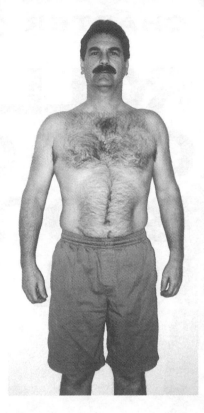

Sam after

Nicolas before

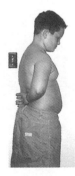

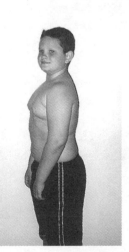

Nicolas after

Carrie before

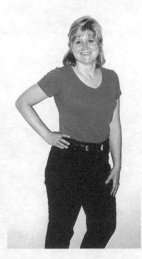

Carrie after

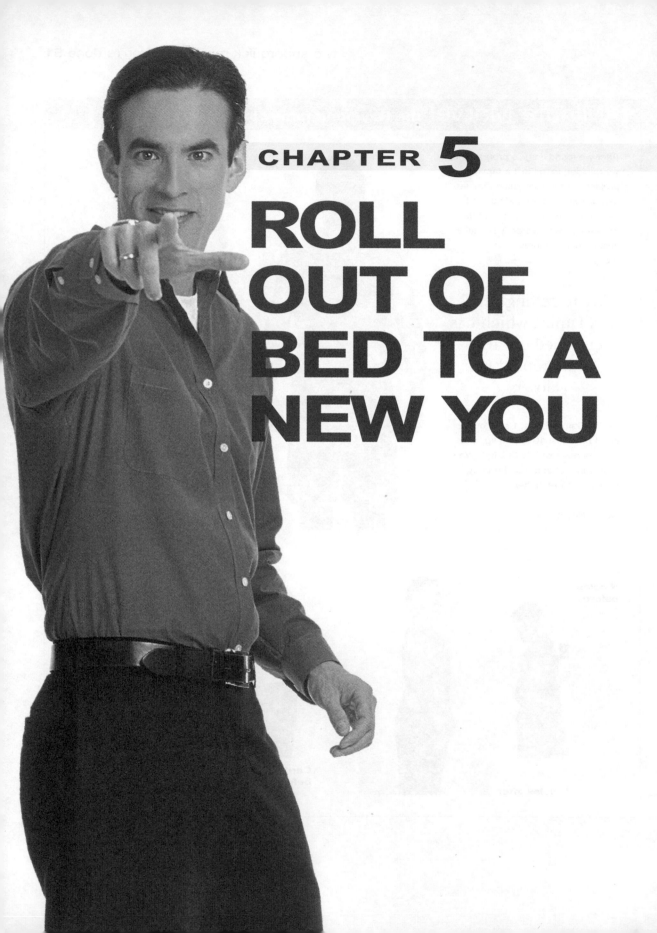

CHAPTER 5

ROLL OUT OF BED TO A NEW YOU

why move in the morning?

When I suggest to people that they get up 8 minutes earlier in the morning to exercise, I sometimes get: 'Oh, I'm not a morning person. That will never work for me. As soon as the alarm goes off, I'll hit the snooze button.' If you keep thinking that way, that's what you'll do.

'There's no such thing as not being a morning person.'

I truly believe that there's no such thing as not being a morning person; that's all in your head. I used to stay up late at night because I thought of myself as a night owl. Our thoughts are powerful, and they control our actions. I would read, watch television, listen to music and talk to friends on the phone. So when I first started exercising in the morning, I had a really tough time doing it consistently. It's hard to get out of bed in the morning when you only crawled *into* bed a few hours before.

But I was motivated to turn things around. I only had to remind myself of Dad's bout with prostate cancer, my grandmother's death from a stroke and Grandpa's scare with

8 minute marvel Lisa lost 17 lb (7.7 kg)!

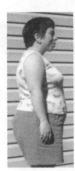
before

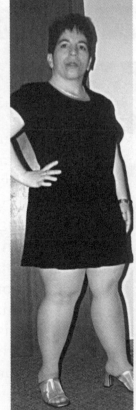
after
A couple of weeks is all it took Lisa to lose weight and increase her energy

'Once I got started, I just wanted to do more. It's great to want to walk up the stairs or to the corner shop rather than drive.'

high blood pressure to motivate myself to get a proper night's sleep. And when I exercised in the morning, I felt wonderful for the rest of the day. Now I don't stay up later than 10 p.m, and I'm out of bed by 6 in the morning.

rise and shine

Consider the case of Lisa Kasirye, one of my online clients. She works from 9.30 a.m. to 6 p.m. After work, she cooks, cleans and sometimes attends night classes. When I first met Lisa, she didn't even start thinking about getting ready for bed until after 10 p.m. At the beginning of her programme, she told me that she slept exhaustedly until 8.30 every morning. She slept away most of her weekends. She couldn't imagine a good reason for getting up any earlier.

But then Lisa committed to 8 Minutes in the Morning. At first, she got up only 15 minutes earlier than usual. After only a couple of weeks on the programme, she had lost weight and her energy level had skyrocketed. 'I have the energy to work out *and* go walking. I enjoy it! This incredible energy is something I never dreamed of. I'm so revitalized that I want to participate in life to the fullest,' she told me.

After 9 weeks on the programme, she had lost 17 lb (7.7 kg). 'Once I got started, I just wanted to do more. It's great to want to walk up the stairs or walk to the corner shop rather than drive,' she said.

If you think Lisa is an exception, think again. My programme affected Howard Joseph the same way.

Howard worked 12- to 14-hour shifts as a professional nurse. He also volunteered his time to mentor secondary school students. Howard, who weighed 22 st (140 kg), didn't have a lot of free time; he had to exercise in the morning or not at all.

He began waking up a few minutes earlier each day to do his 8 Minutes in the Morning exercises. Being on my programme, he lost more than 6 st (41 kg), changed his diet, turned his bedroom into an

---

8 minute marvel Howard lost 91 lb (41 kg)

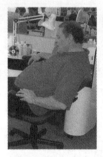

before

after
Turning his bedroom into an exercise room and getting up early have paid dividends for Howard.

'For me, the programme creates wonderful results without struggle. I indulge in chocolate on occasion – my fat-burning metabolism easily burns the extra calories.'

exercise room, and began getting up at 4.30 a.m. to do his exercises, followed by 4 or more miles of powerwalking. 'The morning exercises are great, and the effect really accumulates,' Howard said. 'For me, the morning exercise programme creates wonderful results without struggle.'

morning benefits

When people ask me if they can do their 8 Minutes at any time of the day, I tell them that they will miss out on three major benefits. Exercising in the morning will:

• Boost your metabolism – BOOST!
• Let you maintain consistency – MAINTAIN!
• Allow you to enjoy your weight-loss journey – ENJOY!

When you first wake up in the morning, your metabolism is sluggish because it has slowed down during sleep. When you exercise, your metabolism increases. Thus, exercising in the morning enhances your metabolism when it's naturally the slowest.

The bottom line is that physiologically you burn more fat when you exercise in the morning, making better use of

Without struggle! Another one of my clients, Joseph Newsome, put it this way: 'The morning exercises get my day started and leave me feeling great. My energy has risen to a level that I cannot ever remember having. I start my day feeling pumped up!'

your exercise time. Morning is the only time of day that most people can control. Later in the day, distractions will come up. Things that demand your time –

your questions

What if my workouts take longer than 8 minutes?

Don't worry. Once you get the hang of the exercises and routine, they will go even faster. You should take about 1 minute to perform one set of 12 repetitions of an exercise. The key is to immediately move to the second exercise. Do this for a total of four sets, and you should be done in 8 minutes.

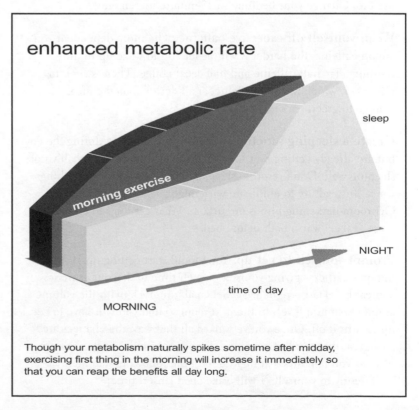

enhanced metabolic rate

sleep

morning exercise

NIGHT

time of day

MORNING

Though your metabolism naturally spikes sometime after midday, exercising first thing in the morning will increase it immediately so that you can reap the benefits all day long.

including your partner, your children, your job – will interrupt your schedule. You may plan to do your exercises during a lunch break, but a friend asks you to lunch and you think, 'OK, I'll do them after work.' But after work, your 10-year-old asks for help with his homework. Then your partner wants to snuggle up on the sofa.

Morning vs. Evening

A 500-person study conducted at the Mollen Clinic in Phoenix, Arizona, showed that only 25 per cent of evening exercisers consistently do their exercise routines, compared to 75 per cent of morning exercisers. The bottom line is that when you commit to exercising in the morning, you bypass excuses and get the fat off faster. The clinic's founder, Dr Art Mollen, says that 'as the day goes on, people pull out the bow and arrows and hunt for excuses not to exercise – like having to work a bit later, run errands, or go out with friends'.

In a study at the University of Leeds, researchers found that women who worked out in the morning reported less tension and greater feelings of contentment than those who didn't exercise in the morning. Exercising sends a signal to your pituitary gland to release endorphins, your body's natural feel-good drug, first thing in the day. The more endorphins you have in your bloodstream, the better you feel. When you exercise in the morning, you will feel and handle yourself better no matter what happens in your day, whether it's getting stuck in a traffic jam, dealing with an annoying colleague or tending to a sick child.

---

sleep secrets

As you progress through the 8 Minutes in the Morning programme, getting out of bed will become easier and easier because you'll start looking forward to your exercises. Be patient: as you lose weight and become more fit, your energy level will grow! Here are a few tips to help you get through the first week.

Take baby steps. Your body has a set internal clock, and you'll have a hard time falling asleep an hour or more earlier than you're used to. Change your bedtime in 15-minute increments.

Wean yourself off excessive caffeine. The more dependent you are on caffeine, the harder it will be for you to wake up in the morning. Try half-caffeine and half-decaf coffee. Then, switch to either tea, which has less caffeine, or all-decaffeinated coffee. Then change to green tea or decaffeinated tea.

Create a sleeping sanctuary. If you often feel tired during the day but are already getting 8 or more hours of sleep, you're probably not sleeping well. Don't resort to sleeping pills: they'll just make things worse. Instead, try to eliminate what might be keeping you awake. Get room-darkening blinds or curtains. Wear earplugs to eliminate noise. Take a warm bath before bed.

Prompt yourself to get up. You should start getting up 10 to 15 minutes earlier – giving yourself enough time to do your exercises and eat breakfast – right away. Set an alarm clock (with the volume at the maximum level) in the next room so that you will have to get up to turn it off. Once you've walked all that way, the chances are very great that you'll stay up and do your 8 Minutes in the Morning. Also, as you fall asleep at night, repeat the following statement confidently to yourself: 'I will wake up at [insert time].'

Additional Morning Benefits

There are other benefits to morning exercise to consider. First, a study at Indiana University suggests that morning workouts reduce blood pressure. In fact, morning exercisers experienced an 8-point drop in systolic pressure (top number) that lasted 11 hours. Their diastolic pressure (bottom number) dropped 6 points for up to 4 hours after exercise. Evening exercisers showed no significant reductions.

There is some evidence, according to the American College of Sports Medicine, that confirms that hormonal responses to strength training are strongest in the morning. Resting levels of testosterone, the body's primary muscle-building hormone, are highest in the morning.

In addition, following a bout of resistance training, testosterone elevations are more marked in the morning compared to the afternoon or early evening. This suggests that the muscle-building potential of strength training may be at its peak before noon.

The bottom line is that exercising is the ultimate endorphin booster and your ultimate advantage to enjoying your new lifestyle. You'll feel healthy after your morning sessions, which will help you focus on your Eat Fat to Get Fit eating plan and help motivate you each step of the way.

sleep: repair muscles and get firmer

Most people have trouble waking up in the morning because they don't get enough sleep at night. On average, most people get at least an hour too little sleep on a regular basis.

In addition to diet and exercise, sleep is one of the most important components of a long and healthy life. If you get too little sleep, you eat more just to stay awake. Plus studies show that lack of sleep also can slow your metabolism, preventing your body from using glucose effectively.

Lack of sleep also affects your levels of leptin, the hormone that makes you feel full. When levels are low, you crave sweets, desserts and even starches.

But the worst effects of sleep deprivation have to do with growth hormone levels. Growth hormone affects your body's proportion of fat to muscle as well as repairs muscles while you sleep.

If you don't get enough sleep at night, your daily exercise session will feel harder than it should. You'll have a harder time building muscle and keeping fat at bay.

You have to promise yourself that you will really start going to bed earlier. It will help you wake up earlier and lose weight faster. It's that important to you.

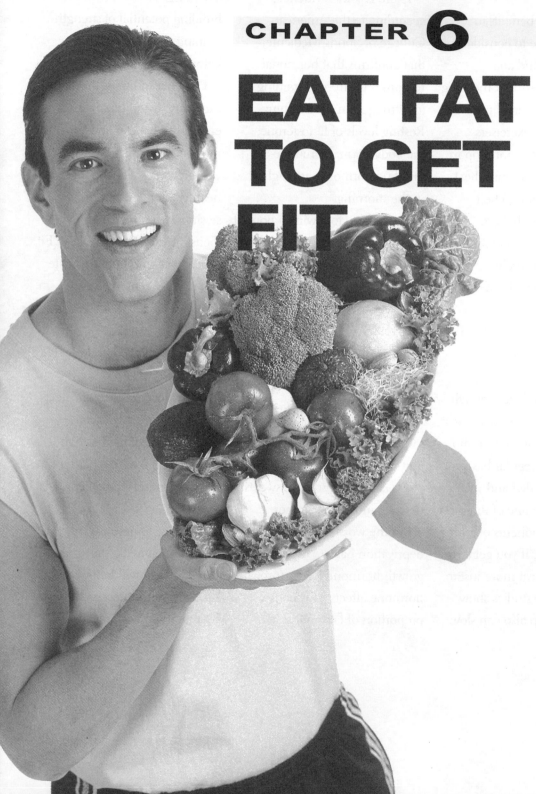

CHAPTER 6

EAT FAT TO GET FIT

bring back the joy of eating and lose more weight

To get the results you want, you must combine your 8 Minutes in the Morning exercise routine with my Eat Fat to Get Fit Eating Card System. You heard right . . . eat fat! A simple little three-letter word, fat is too often overlooked when people are trying to lose weight. Most of us have been programmed to believe that all fats are bad and will only make us fatter. But we have been misled. It is essential for you to know that *eating a fat-free diet is the worst thing you can do when you want to lose weight!*

fat

I have broken the programme down into seven different food groups: Fat, Protein, Complex Carbohydrates, Dairy, Vegetables, Fruit and Treats and Cravings. With each food group broken down, it is very simple to monitor what you eat if you follow the Eating Card System (see page 74). The Eating Cards will help you know that you have got all of the right foods in your body and the good and bad characteristics of each. The more you understand what you

eat and why, the better choices you will make. (And, as always, you must drink water – no less than eight glasses a day.)

Certain fats are considered 'good' fats and, when eaten with your meals, are critical to maximizing your weight loss. There are three amazing ways that these good fats will help you lose weight. They:
- Are the ultimate appetite suppressant – SUPPRESS!
- Help unlock stored body fat – UNLOCK!

- Boost your body's metabolic rate, helping you to burn more body fat – BURN!

Think of it as a mantra: 'Suppress, unlock and burn!' (Like 'Boost, maintain and enjoy!' on page 55.) This is how you will Eat Fat to Get Fit. Read on to see why low-fat and fat-free diets are not the answer, then find out what the good fats are, how they work exactly and where you can get them.

The Big Fat Misunderstanding

Over the past decade, fat has earned a bad reputation. Magazine articles, food marketers and even weight-loss experts have told us that all fats are bad and that eating any type of fat will make you fat. This thinking promoted and perpetuated the no-fat craze, and food companies have made millions of pounds from it. Just visit the supermarket and look at all the fat-free versions of your favourite foods in one aisle after another.

Oddly enough, throughout this entire no-fat craze, people continued to get fatter. They bought fat-free crisps, cakes and biscuits but their waistlines expanded. How could that happen? For one, to make fat-free foods taste good, manufacturers had to add more sugar. Essentially, by the time they had created the fat-free version of the biscuit or cheesecake, the product had just as many calories as the higher-fat version.

Scientists once thought that if you cut fat out of your diet, you would lose weight. They based this thinking on a number of factors, including that 1 gram of fat equals 9 calories, whereas 1 gram of carbohydrate or protein equals just 4. Coupled with that was the misconception that all dietary fat is converted to body fat more easily than carbohydrates or proteins. This led people to believe that they could only gain weight by eating fat, and that they could eat as much as they wanted all the time, as long as it was fat-free.

avoid the fat trap

To avoid fattening, unhealthy fats, you need to understand what types of foods they hide in. Here are some examples for two specific types of bad fats.

Saturated fats. Found in high amounts in animal products such as beef, lamb, bacon, pâté, salami, sausages, cheese, butter and cream. You can avoid these fats – and continue to eat animal products – if you:

- Choose lower-fat options such as the white meat of chicken and turkey without the skin and reduced-fat dairy products. Even with red meat, look for the lowest-fat options (extra-lean mince, fillet and rump steak, trimmed of fat, lean bacon, ham and venison). I also recommend that you try soya versions of meat products – they taste great and are much more healthy.

- Watch your portion size. Think of meat and dairy products as condiments, not as your main course. Restrict yourself to a 3- to 6-oz (90- to 70-g) serving of meat a day, roughly the size of one to two packs of cards. My Eating Card System will help you stay on track.

Trans fats. Also called hydrogenated fats, trans fats have no physical purpose in your body. They are a type of fat you could cut completely out of your diet and your body would not notice the difference. These fats are made when foods are processed, so they can be found in just about everything that has been packaged or changed from its natural state. Common trans fat culprits include biscuits, cakes, ready-made pastry, doughnuts, muffins, margarine and many spreads, crisps, crackers and savoury snacks.

The Fear of Fats

I'm sure most of you are thinking the same thing: 'Wait a minute! If I include more fat in my diet, I am just going to get fatter!' Although fat does have nearly double the calories of carbohydrates and proteins, not all calories – and certainly not all fats – are created equally.

Some fats are not good for you and are converted to body fat faster, especially those that are saturated, hydrogenated, fried or heat-processed. Found in red meat, butter, margarine, fried chicken and doughnuts, these fats tend to trigger eating episodes. (Don't worry, you can still eat these foods. I will show you how.) If you've ever had one, you know exactly what I'm talking about. A colleague brings in a box of doughnuts. You decide that you'll have one to make her feel good. Suddenly, you've eaten not one but two doughnuts as well as a bag of crisps.

Studies show that these types of fats are indeed addictive, making you want to eat more. They are also incredibly bad for your health. Saturated and hydrogenated fats have been linked to just about every health condition from heart disease to diabetes to cancer.

I do not recommend these fats in my Eat Fat to Get Fit programme, but you can have them in moderation. More important, you will discover the good fats, the fats that I want you to incorporate into all your meals. These are called *omega fats*, and they'll help you get lean while making your food taste great.

What exactly are omega fats? They are sometimes called essential fatty acids (EFAs), because they are fats your body

eat fat to get fit: quick reference chart

Omega-3. Get it from liquid flax oil (make this the primary fat that you add to your meals). Use it on salads or bread, and add it to soups (after cooking) and yoghurt. Do not cook with this fat.

Omega-6. You get omega-6 fats from pre-packaged foods like crisps and shop-bought foods. You get enough of this fat, so avoid adding it to your meals.

Omega-9. Olive oil, avocados, peanuts, almonds and macadamia nuts all include omega-9 fats. It's the second-best oil to add to your meals because it enhances your use of omega-3 fat. Olive oil should be your number-one cooking fat. When eating out in restaurants, ask for olive oil to use on your salad instead of dressing and dip your bread into it instead of using butter.

cannot make and must have for optimum performance. They are almost never stored as fat because they are used by your body in maintaining healthy cell membranes, brain function, healthy skin, strong hair and strong nails, and are directly related to thousands of life-sustaining metabolic functions.

Three of the most well-known and well-researched omega fats are the omega-3s, omega-6s, and omega-9s. Though omega-9 fats are not considered essential, they are still critical because they enhance the benefits of the omega-3s. I strongly recommend that you include all three types of omega fats in your meal plan.

So how do omega fats get you slim? As I shared with you at the beginning of this chapter, there are three amazing weight-loss benefits to using omega fats.

Suppress Appetite

Probably the most powerful benefit that omega fats give you is that they are the ultimate appetite suppressant. By adding omega fats to your foods or taking them with a meal, you will have a strong feeling of satiety, fullness and satisfaction. Omega fats cause the stomach to retain food for a longer period of time as compared to fat-free or low-fat foods. That's because fats require greater digestive energy than proteins and carbohydrates. As a result, they are held in the stomach longer than other food sources, and they help to stimulate the release of cholecystokinin (CCK), a gut hormone that signals the brain to stop eating. According to studies done at Pennsylvania State University and Thomas Jefferson University – Jefferson Medical College, in Philadelphia, of all the nutrients you can eat, omega fats do the best job of promoting the feeling of fullness and satiety. In other words, you require smaller meals to make you feel satisfied, and you stay satisfied for longer periods of time – up to 6 hours.

My good friend Jade Beutler, author of two wonderful books, *Understanding Fats and Oils* and *Flax for Life*, shared with me a great metaphor that I will never forget. He says that when you eat omega fats, you can think of yourself as a super-efficient car, getting 30 miles per gallon of petrol; as opposed to a fuel hog that is getting 10 miles per gallon (when you eat fat-free). The fuel hog uses more fuel more quickly and therefore has to stop more frequently at the pump (or fridge) to fill up. But by eating your meals with omega fats, you automatically get better 'mileage'.

And that's the ticket. You will feel fuller longer and not experience hunger pangs or the desire to snack between meals.

Unlock Stored Body Fat

Eating the right amounts of omega fats helps to *unlock stored body fat so that you can better use it as energy*. Omega fat balances your body's ratio of insulin to glucagon. When you eat sugary foods, your body secretes the hormone insulin to remove the excess sugar from your body. When you eat excessively sugary meals, your body releases too much insulin, blocking the critical pancreatic hormone glucagon from operating effectively within your body. Glucagon is a key hormone that enables your body to burn its stores of body fat. A diet rich in omega fats helps balance your insulin levels so that glucagon can be released to unlock your body's fat-storage banks and begin converting unwanted body fat into energy.

Burn Body Fat

Omega fats boost your body's metabolic rate, which in turn helps you burn more body fat! No other fat on Earth will do this. Your metabolic rate will increase in two natural and healthy ways. Your body will immediately utilize the omega fats to maintain the integrity and function of your body's 75 trillion cell membranes. Having healthier cell membranes means that you improve the 'vehicles' that transport oxygen, one of the key elements in everyday fat burning. The more oxygen you have available, the easier it is for your lean muscle tissue to convert body fat into the energy it needs to sustain itself.

The body fat you want to burn, called white fat, lies near the top of your skin. There is another type of fat, called brown fat, that lies deep within your body and surrounds your vital organs – your heart, kidneys and adrenal glands. It also cushions your spinal column as well as your neck and major thoracic blood vessels.

By *activating* your brown fat, your body will burn more calories for heat rather than retaining those calories for future use. Brown fat is not a storage fat like white fat, but rather a calorie-burning engine. Ann Louise Gittleman, MS, CNS, one of the foremost nutritionists in the United States, explains that 'although brown fat makes up 10 per cent or less of total body fat, it is responsible for 25 per cent of all the fat calories burned by all the other body tissues'. So having a second type of fat-burning furnace is almost like having more lean muscle tissue!

Still not convinced that you can Eat Fat to Get Fit . . . that you will lose weight and look great? Just read what a few of my clients have to say about adding omega fats to their diets.

- 'I spent months eating low-fat foods and doing 60 minutes of high-impact aerobics every day and got nowhere. When I was unable to fit into my pre-pregnancy clothes after 2 years, I became depressed,' says Stephanie Donald. 'When I started to Eat Fat to Get Fit, I weighed 11½ st (73 kg) and had a 31-inch (78-cm) waist. After 8 weeks, I had lost a stone (6.4 kg) in weight and 2 inches (5 cm) from my waist!'
- 'I do not feel like I'm in food prison with many restrictions and limitations,' says former emotional eater Howard Joseph.
- 'Adding omega fats to my diet made me feel satisfied,' says

Amber Dunlap. 'I don't feel moody as I did with other diets that I've tried. I really like that I am eating enough for my body, and I can feel the difference. The fat is melting off! This is the easiest weight I have ever lost!'

Good for Your Health, Too

The Eat Fat to Get Fit programme not only helps you shed weight but also helps you live longer. The unappreciated good guys for a number of years, omega fats have only relatively recently received the respect they deserve. Quite a bit of research has been done that supports the idea of using omega fats to help you reach your weight-loss goal as well as improve your overall health.

- A study completed in the United Kingdom found that supplementing with omega fats – not saturated fats or even polyunsaturated fats – changed the composition of joint cartilage, reducing the pain and inflammation associated with various types of arthritis. Another study found that patients who took omega fat supplements were able to

omega fats = good fats

Though any fat can help satisfy your appetite or even release stored body fat, omega fats, particularly omega-3s, offer a number of uniquely wonderful benefits.

- They cannot ever be converted into the 'bad' saturated fats. This is important because excessive intake of saturated fat is closely linked to obesity, cancer, heart disease, stroke and premature death. Hundreds of research studies show that omega fats can actually help prevent all these things, plus certain types of diabetes.
- In women, omega fats have been shown to help ease premenstrual syndrome and postmenopausal discomfort.
- In men, omega fats have been shown to improve sex drive.

completely stop taking their anti-inflammatory painkillers for arthritic disease.
- A study from Korea found that people who eat more omega fats on a daily basis experience a lower risk of prostate cancer and prostate inflammation. Numerous other studies have shown a decreased risk for other types of cancers as well.

- A study done in the Netherlands found that supplementing with omega fats reduced some of the intestinal inflammation associated with Crohn's disease. Many other studies have shown that diets high in omega fats reduce all sorts of gastrointestinal problems, from chronic diarrhoea to chronic constipation.
- Research strongly shows that increasing the omega fats in your diet while simultaneously decreasing the saturated and trans fats can boost immunity, regulate blood sugar, prevent diabetes, reduce heart disease and stroke, treat asthma, lift depression, prevent Alzheimer's disease and, of course, promote weight loss.

Here are some tips to help you get more healthy good fats into your diet.

- Although cold-water fish such as salmon and mackerel are higher in protein than they are in fat, they do contain enough omega-3 fatty acids to deserve a mention here. Since fish is not a superconcentrated source of omega fats, you will only cross off Protein boxes, not Fat boxes on your Eating Cards. It is great for lunch or dinner.
- If you like butter, you can make your own healthy butter substitute. Pour extra-virgin olive oil (omega-9 fat) into a plastic airtight container and then cover. Refrigerate it overnight to harden it. Then you can spread it just as you would butter!
- Going nuts for a great midday snack? Try almonds. These healthy nuts make a perfect snack because they are packed full of omega-9 fats and will help you burn fat while satisfying your midday hunger pangs. Other omega-packed nuts include hazelnuts, pecans, macadamia nuts and pistachios.
- Eat avocados. These green, pear-shaped foods taste so delicious that it's hard to believe they are good for you. Avocado makes a great spread on wholemeal toast instead of sugary jam. It's great to add to any salad. A ripe avocado is slightly soft – not hard – to your touch.
- Use olive oil in place of salad dressing on your salad or when you don't have flax oil available.

try this at home

In a zip-up plastic bag, put 3 teaspoons of butter, a traditional saturated fat. In another bag, pour 3 teaspoons of olive oil (primarily omega-9). In a third bag, pour 3 teaspoons of liquid flax oil (primarily omega-3). Then seal the bags and put them in the refrigerator overnight. The next morning, you'll see that both the butter and olive oil have hardened in the cold. Only the flax oil will have remained liquid. Flax oil is the least saturated oil in the world, making it the body's favourite to use (not store) and the ideal choice for weight loss.

The Best Slimming Omega Source

The best omega fat source for weight loss is one that is the richest in omega-3 fat. Why omega-3, and not omega-6 or omega-9? Omega-3 fat is the least saturated fat – the most pliable and non-solid. That means that omega-3 fat is the body's top choice for maintaining everything from healthy cell membranes to brain function. When your body uses the omega-3 fats for these types of necessary bodily functions, there is literally no more of it left

FINDING THE FRIENDLY FATS

Where is the best place to find omega-3 fat? Check out the chart below to see which source is the best choice. Fresh flax oil is the winner, with a whopping 57 per cent of the precious omega-3 fat.

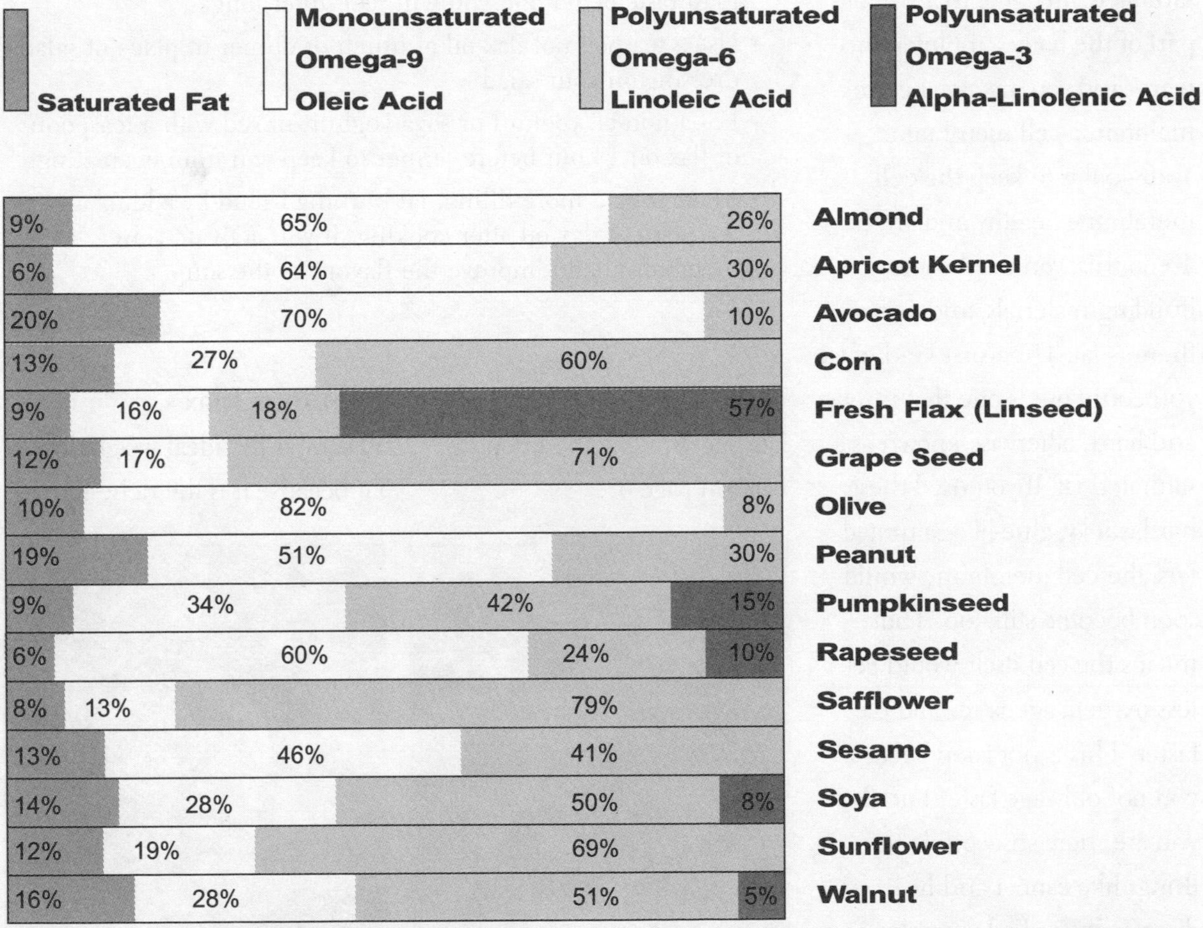

	Saturated Fat	Monounsaturated Omega-9 Oleic Acid	Polyunsaturated Omega-6 Linoleic Acid	Polyunsaturated Omega-3 Alpha-Linolenic Acid
Almond	9%	65%	26%	
Apricot Kernel	6%	64%	30%	
Avocado	20%	70%	10%	
Corn	13%	27%	60%	
Fresh Flax (Linseed)	9%	16%	18%	57%
Grape Seed	12%	17%	71%	
Olive	10%	82%	8%	
Peanut	19%	51%	30%	
Pumpkinseed	9%	34%	42%	15%
Rapeseed	6%	60%	24%	10%
Safflower	8%	13%	79%	
Sesame	13%	46%	41%	
Soya	14%	28%	50%	8%
Sunflower	12%	19%	69%	
Walnut	16%	28%	51%	5%

Source: NatureMed Research, Inc.

to be stored on your body as body fat.

Why does your body better utilize a fat that is the least saturated, such as omega-3 fat rather than a fat that is more saturated? Imagine that you are part of the body's 'maintenance team' and you are assigned to maintain a cell membrane. Your goal is to keep the cell membrane healthy and alive. To do this, you need some building materials, and one of them is fat. The worst kind of fat you could use is one that is solid and hard, otherwise known as a saturated fat. If you used these hard, sticky, glue-like saturated fats, the cell membrane would soon become stiff, too. That means the cell itself would get less oxygen, age faster and die faster. This is not good because you not only age faster but also you are more susceptible to things like cancer and heart disease. If you had your choice, you would select the least saturated fat possible, and that would be an omega-3 fat, followed by omega-6 and omega-9 respectively. Just remember, the lower the number, the better the fat is for you. The higher the number, the more saturated it is.

how to 'flaxize' your meals

Here are a few tips to easily add flax oil into your meals. If you want to share your great ideas for getting more flax into your diet, e-mail them to *flaxsize@jorgecruise.com*.

- Instead of a sugary jam spread on your toast in the morning, use flax oil (pretend it is melted butter). It will make your toast taste better and you will feel fuller longer.
- Use a teaspoon of flax oil at lunch or dinner in place of salad dressing on your salad.
- Eat a non-fat yoghurt or soya yoghurt mixed with a teaspoon of flax oil 1 hour before dinner to keep you from overeating.
- Make soup a more filling, fat-burning friend by adding a teaspoon of flax oil after cooking. It will activate your metabolism and improve the flavour of the soup.

For a comparison of the omega fats, see 'Finding the Friendly Fats' on page 65.

Fabulous Flax

Flax oil is the ideal weight-loss fat because it is the richest

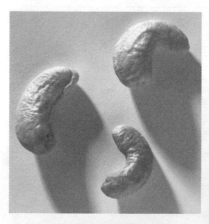
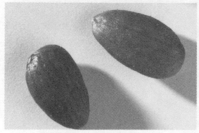
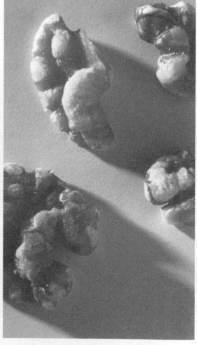

Eating more omega fats will help you eat less, enjoy your food, boost your metabolism, avoid disease and feel happier.

source of omega-3 fats. Plus, it has the ideal amount of omega-6 and omega-9. You get omega-6 from things like safflower, sunflower, soya bean and corn oils, which are used in many pre-packaged foods. So, most of us are getting plenty of omega-6 already. What you need to focus on is getting more omega-3s into your diet with flax. Flax also contains omega-9, and though it's not essential, the positive effects of the Mediterranean diet are largely attributed to omega-9 fatty acids. The bottom line is that flax oil has a perfect blend of all three omega fats to help you lose weight!

Flax oil comes from flaxseeds, also called linseeds. I recommend that you buy flax in liquid form because it is the most efficient. The oil is made by cold-pressing thousands of seeds to extract the oil. The oil is immediately refrigerated to preserve its freshness. You can use the liquid form directly on your foods, and this is where the flavour and fun starts. Think of it as a great flavour-enhancing condiment you can use with all your meals. I use it during breakfast on toast, at lunch I put

it on my salad, and at dinner I use it on my brown rice or steamed veggies. Liquid flax oil can be found in all health food stores. And for those of you who travel or just don't like the taste of fat, you can get flax oil in capsule form too.

Just how important is supplementing your diet with flax oil? I am such a big believer in the weight-loss power of flax, I personally use it every day. For more information on Jorge Cruise's Weight Loss Secret, visit *www.jorgecruise.com.flax*.

How Much Fat?

I don't want you to think that you can eat only omega fats on this programme. You can still enjoy a variety of fats with your meals, even saturated fats like butter, and you can still use corn oil or whatever other oils you like – just use them in moderation. A complete list of all the fats you can use on this programme appears on page 214.

The amount of fat you need depends on your current weight and caloric needs. Don't worry. You don't need to spend any time with a calculator and chart to work out how much fat to eat

the right portions

To cross off the right number of boxes in your Eating Card System, you have to know how much you are eating. But you don't need to measure and weigh everything you eat. Here are some simple examples of how to approximately gauge your food portions by comparing them to the size of parts of your hand.

Thumb tip. 1 box of olive oil, flax oil or avocado

Fist. 1 box of green vegetables, grains or whole fruit

Cupped hand. 1 box of dairy

Palm of hand (excluding fingers and thumb). 3 boxes of protein

in a day. I've done all the work for you. As long as you use your Eating Card System, you will automatically eat the right amount and right types of fat at every meal.

I've also assembled an easy-to-use general Food List (see page 214) that will help you make smart choices and cross off the correct boxes with your Eating Card System (see page 74).

protein

Have you ever lost a significant amount of weight on a diet, only to plateau well before you reached your goal? That's probably because you weren't eating enough protein. Sometimes eating more helps you lose more weight.

Protein is your body's building material. You need to eat protein to provide your body with the materials it needs to build, repair and maintain your lean muscle tissue. That's incredibly important because without enough dietary protein, all of your 8 Minutes in the Morning moves will be for nothing. And over half of your body weight is made up of protein. This includes not only muscle tissue but also hair, skin, nails, blood, hormones, enzymes, brain cells and much more.

When you don't eat enough protein, your body actually starts to break down and recycle existing body protein (such as lean muscle) to supply your body with the amino acids that your diet is lacking. When this protein breakdown occurs, you sacrifice muscle (your fat-burning machine) and your metabolism slows down. As a result, you burn less body fat.

Protein is important, but don't go overboard. You've probably heard about – and may have even tried – one of the popular high-protein diets. When I interviewed best-selling author Dr Andrew Weil, for my *FitNow.com* online television show, he shared with me what's wrong with these diets: they work for weight loss – temporarily – because you're eating more protein than your body needs to repair tissue, and your body burns the excess as fuel. Unfortunately, protein is a 'dirty' source of fuel because it contains nitrogen. Instead of producing just carbon dioxide and water,

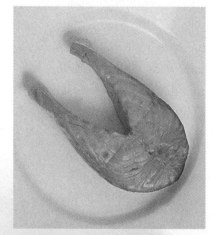

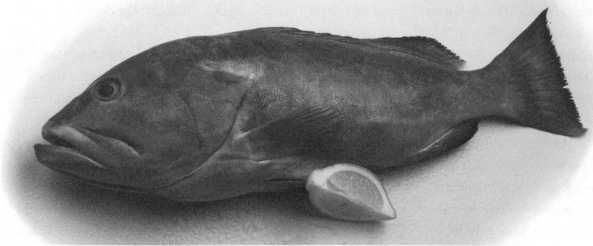

Eating more of the right types of protein will help you build calorie-hungry muscle, boost your metabolism, and feel less hungry.

protein produces nitrogenous residues, which are toxic. Your body must pump a lot of water into the urinary tract to flush the toxic nitrogen out. In other words, much of the 'weight loss' from high-protein diets is simply water loss. While this is going on, you're also losing minerals from your body, including calcium from your bones.

To eat the right amount of protein, all you need to do is follow your Eating Card System and consult the Food List on page 214 for the best sources.

Besides getting protein in the right amounts, you also want to focus on the right types. Some types of protein – especially the type found in animal products – contain a high amount of saturated fat, which can not only hinder your weight-loss efforts but also destroy your health. Focus on high-quality protein sources like fish, skinless white-meat chicken and turkey, soya products, egg whites, legumes and beans.

Soya beans are a quality protein source that is naturally low in saturated fat. If you're a vegetarian, eating soya is the best way to ensure that you consume all of the amino acids you need.

Even if you're not a vegetarian, I recommend adding soya to your diet because it has been shown to reduce heart disease, cancer, osteoporosis, menopausal symptoms and more. You'll find it in veggie versions of burgers, hot dogs, 'bacon' and cheeses as well as in tofu, miso, soya milk and soya nuts. Tofu is a great meat extender. Mix it with meat or cheese to lower the saturated fat in your recipes.

When you have a hankering for red meat, go ahead and have it, but choose lean sirloin, fillet or topside, eat a small portion, and trim off any visible fat. Limit your red meat consumption to no more than twice a week. Beef comes marbled with non-essential fat that is mostly saturated. It is the worst animal fat in terms of chemical composition, containing 51 per cent saturated fatty acids (SFAs). In comparison, pig lard, still very bad, has 41 per cent SFAs.

complex carbohydrates

My Eat Fat to Get Fit programme includes carbohydrates because they play a critical role in achieving fat loss. You read it right: carbohydrates can be used to get you lean. The key is to avoid simple carbohydrates that are

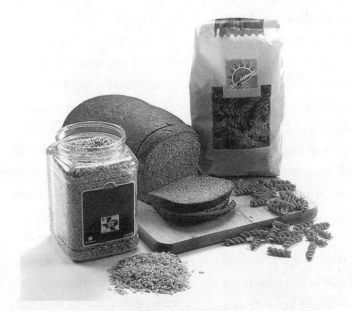

Eating more of the right types of carbohydrates will help you burn more body fat, balance insulin levels, feel less hungry, and prevent disease.

'Complex carbohydrates never overwhelm your body with sugar rushes because they take more time to break down.'

high on the glycaemic index, which rates how fast a particular food turns into glucose (blood sugar), and eat complex carbohydrates that are much lower on the index. The higher the number, the faster it turns into glucose. Simple carbohydrates such as processed white bread and rice release quickly. Complex carbohydrates, on the other hand, are usually whole grain and unprocessed.

How does avoiding simple carbohydrates help you burn body fat? When your insulin is balanced, more of the hormone glucagon is available to help unlock body fat stores. You can help balance insulin levels further by avoiding the foods that drastically increase insulin levels: simple carbohydrates.

Simple vs. Complex

Simple carbohydrates not only prevent you from burning pre-existing body fat but also encourage you to gain more

body fat. When you eat a large meal that is made from simple carbohydrates, you are left with an immediate abundance of glucose, more than your body could ever need or use. Some of the glucose that is not used right away by your muscles is stored in your liver and muscles as glycogen (stored blood sugar). The rest is converted and stored as body fat. This is why you can remain overweight even though you are eating low-fat or fat-free foods.

The solution is to eat complex carbohydrates, which provide you with just the right amount of energy while burning excess body fat. Imagine that you're starting a campfire. You would light the big logs by using lighter fluid or kindling. That's exactly how complex carbohydrates work in your body. Instead of wood, it's body fat. By trickling in small amounts of complex carbohydrates, the fat will burn steadily for a long time. If you

pour too much lighter fluid (simple carbohydrates) on at one time, you get a flash fire that flares quickly and then burns out almost immediately.

Unlike simple carbohydrates, complex carbohydrates are not rapidly released into your bloodstream because of their complex molecular structure. This means that complex carbohydrates never overwhelm your body with sugar rushes because they take more time to break down. They provide the ideal amounts of time-released sugar to burn fat. This allows your body to use body fat as its primary fuel.

To find out which foods are complex carbohydrates and which are simple carbohydrates, consult the Food List on page 214. But you can also use this simple rule of thumb: the more 'whole' or natural a food is, the more likely it is to be complex.

Whole Grains

Whole grains – those that contain their outer shells or husks – are more complex than refined grains, which have been stripped of their outer coatings. In other words, slow-cooking, wholegrain oats are better than instant oats, brown rice is better than white rice, wholegrain bread is better than white bread, and wholewheat pasta is better than regular pasta. Another good rule of thumb is to check the fibre content. Foods that are higher in fibre – with at least 3g or more per 100g – tend to be more 'whole' than foods that lack fibre.

Whole grains are also incredibly good for your health. That outer covering of the grain contains disease-fighting fibre and important phytochemicals. Here are some ways to add different grains to your diet.

• Treat yourself to wholegrain breads from an old-fashioned bakery.

• The slower oatmeal cooks, the more 'whole' it is. Irish oatmeal (also called Scotch or steel-cut oats) is your best source of whole grains. If you don't have time to wait for it to cook on the stove, add it to other recipes, such as meat loaf and stuffing.

• Breakfast cereals are a great source of whole grains if you buy the right kind. The high-sugar, overly processed 'kiddie' cereals are not going to cut it. The better breakfast cereals

contain at least 3g per 100g of fibre and less than 1g per 100g of total fat.

• High in protein and free from gluten, quinoa is a great grain substitute if you are allergic to

dairy foods

Dairy products are supposed to be good for you – their main selling point being that they're high in calcium – but what if you are allergic to them? It was

wheat. It also contains lots of calcium, iron, fibre, B vitamins, vitamin E and folate. It is one of my favourite hot cereals. Add quinoa to soups, stews and cold salads.

after I read *Eating Well for Optimum Health*, an amazing book by Dr Andrew Weil, that my viewpoint on dairy foods changed. The protein found in

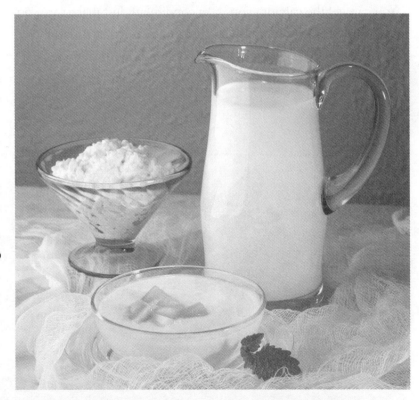

Select healthier versions of dairy products, such as soya, to support your weight loss by reducing sinus problems so that you get more oxygen to burn body fat, boosting your immune system and helping eliminate asthma.

dairy products, called casein, is a known allergen that can cause asthma and sinus problems and can be an irritant to your immune system. Casein has been shown to trigger an autoimmune reaction that destroys insulin-producing cells in the pancreas. That can lead to juvenile diabetes. And digestion of lactose (the sugar in milk) requires the enzyme lactase, which many adults lack. This can cause major digestive distress.

You can get the calcium you need from fortified soya products such as soya milk and soya cheese instead. These are both delicious and healthy alternatives that I use every day. You can also get calcium from fortified juice. Most people don't realize that all green plants – particularly broccoli and kale – have high levels of calcium. And you can always take a calcium supplement.

If you don't have asthma, chronic allergies, hay fever or sinus problems, you can eat traditional dairy products in moderation; I use dairy mostly as a condiment. Just make sure you use products that are low-fat or made from skimmed milk.

your questions

What's your favourite way to make vegetables more exciting to eat?

One of my clients shared this incredibly simple recipe for a tasty veggie dressing. Combine the juice from half a lemon with 1 teaspoon flax oil (1 Fat box) and one crushed garlic clove. Pour over your salad or crudités and enjoy. For more great food ideas, see page 229.

vegetables

Although vegetables are a type of carbohydrate, I've grouped them in their own category because of their unique beneficial effects on fat loss. Vegetables have a very high water content, which means that they are also very high in oxygen. In order for your lean muscle tissue to burn fat, it needs oxygen to help convert the fat into energy. When you eat vegetables, you will flood your body with water, which will dramatically increase your oxygen levels, improving your metabolism.

Vegetables are high in fibre and, ounce for ounce, are probably the most filling low-calorie food you can eat. And

Vegetables are high in water and oxygen, which improves your metabolism; high in fibre, which fills you up; low in simple sugars, which encourages the release of glucagon; low in calories; and high in phytochemicals, which boosts your overall immunity.

since vegetables need to be chewed more and take longer to consume, your brain has time to realize that you are eating and turns off the 'hunger switch' sooner. Once in your stomach, that fibre takes up a lot of space, making you feel full.

Most vegetables are also very low in simple sugars. Vegetables have almost no calories. This means you can literally eat them to your heart's content and not put on excess body fat. For example, to consume a paltry 20 calories, you would have to eat half a cucumber, a whole lettuce, or 6 oz (170 g) of radishes. Besides promoting weight loss, vegetables are superfoods when it comes to your health. They are an important source of vitamins and minerals, and research has shown that brightly coloured vegetables contain substances called phytochemicals that form the plant's immune system. These phytochemicals also act to keep the human immune system strong. In just one serving of green vegetables, more than 100 different phytochemicals may be present to help ward off disease. Think about it. If you are sick less often, you will have more

energy to do the things you love, including sticking to your 8 Minutes in the Morning programme.

You can eat almost all vegetables in unlimited amounts on this programme – that's how low in calories and how good for you they are. Only a few vegetables – especially potatoes and other root vegetables that are high in starch – contain more calories,

and therefore cannot be eaten with abandon (find out which ones on page 218).

Many people are out of the habit of eating vegetables. You want to eat as many servings of green vegetables as you can, particularly when you have a mood-related craving or feel hungry for no apparent reason. See page 229 for some recipes for all-you-can-eat green vegetables.

fruit

You've probably been told that fruit is good for you. But that's true only if you're not trying to lose weight. While fruit does contain a wealth of beneficial nutrients that help your body fight off disease, it also contains high amounts of simple sugars.

Fruit, especially tropical fruit, is high on the glycaemic index. Your body breaks it down and burns it quickly, spiking your insulin levels. High insulin levels block the hormone glucagon, hindering the fat-burning process.

Compared to green vegetables, fruit contains quite a few calories. One banana contains 100 calories. Compare that to 3 oz

(90 g) of asparagus or 3 oz (90 g) of broccoli for only 22 calories.

Fruit is good for you in other ways, so don't cut it completely out of your diet. I suggest limiting yourself to only one serving a day, while pumping up your vegetable servings to six or more. Lemons and limes are the exception; feel free to use them as much as you want. (I love to use lemon or lime in my water every day to help cleanse my body.)

If you love fruit and can't bear the thought of eating only one piece a day, cut your serving in half so that you can eat a small serving of fruit early in the day and another serving later on.

USING THE EATING CARD SYSTEM

The secret to the eating part of my programme is eating the right amount of fat with each meal and monitoring your total food intake. You will do this with your Eating Card System.

Each Eating Card is made up of a series of boxes that represent one selection from the food group. There are seven food groups in my Eat Fat to Get Fit eating plan:

1 Fats
2 Proteins
3 Complex Carbohydrates
4 Dairy
5 Vegetables
6 Fruit
7 Treats and Cravings

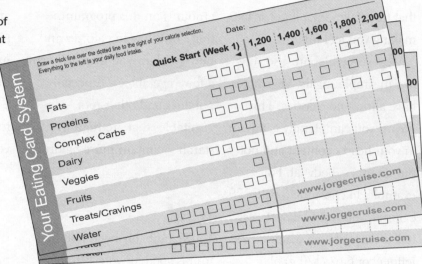

A compete list of recommended foods from each food group is gathered in the Food List on page 214. Each time you eat one portion of food, cross off that box on the card with an X. If you eat three portions, you need to cross off three boxes.

Every time you sit down for a meal or snack, first go to the Food List and decide what you want to eat. Then look at how many boxes that food item uses. Each box equals one portion. The Food List indicates that 3 oz (90 g) cooked pasta is one portion. Therefore, 6 oz (70 g) of cooked pasta would equal two portions; you would cross off 2 Complex Carbohydrate boxes. There is also a place on your

card to cross off eight daily glasses of water. Be sure to drink all of them.

When you finish crossing off all the boxes, you have finished eating for the day. The key is to make sure to eat all the food on your daily Eating Card. Some people think that they can hurry weight loss along by eating even less food than they are allowed on the card. That's dangerous because eating less will generate weight loss from muscle tissue, not just body fat. You must eat all of your food.

If you're still hungry after crossing off all of your boxes, refer to the Food List for the

vegetables that you can eat without limit.

ABOUT THE CARDS

You'll see that I've included master Eating Cards on page 235. The Eating Cards are designed to be photocopied, ideally onto card stock. There are two of the same cards on the page. Make four copies, which gives you enough cards for 7 days plus an extra card. After you photocopy them, cut the cards down the middle and stack them. You can also staple them together to make a booklet. This is now your eating guide for the week. Take it with you everywhere you go. Imagine it's an eating 'chequebook'.

THE FIRST WEEK

For the first week, you will use the Quick Start portion of the Eating Card no matter what your current weight or goal. It's an eating plan that will cleanse your body and help you break your poor eating habits (see A Week of Eating Fat to Get Fit on page 226). It is essential that you follow it precisely. Look at it as a special time to start afresh. After the first week, you will feel great physically. So, to start, draw a thick line over the dotted line to the right of the Quick Start section. All the boxes to the left of this line represent how much you will eat each day of Week 1.

WEEKS 2, 3, 4, AND BEYOND

calorie intake chart

Your current weight lb (kg)	Calories for Women	Calories for Men
10 st 10 lb (68 kg)	1,200	1,400
10 st 10 lb–14 st 3 lb (68–90 kg)	1,400	1,600
14 st 4 lb–17 st 11 lb (91–113 kg)	1,600	1,800
17 st 12 lb–21 st 5 lb (114–136 kg)	2,000	2,000
21 st 6 lb + (137 kg +)	For every 50 lb (22 kg) above 300, add 1 Complex Carbohydrate selection and 1 Protein selection to the 2,000-Calorie section	For every 50 lb (22 kg) above 300, add 1 Complex Carbohydrate selection and 1 Protein selection to the 2,000-Calorie section

For the remainder of the programme, select the calorie intake that is right for you. How do you know which to use after Week 1? For now, you will be using your gender and current weight as a guide. As your weight goes down, you will move to the next calorie selection to continue your fat burning. For example, if you are a woman who weighs 13 st 8 lb (86 kg), you will use the 1,400 Calories section. When you reach 10 st 9 lb (68 kg), you will change to the 1,200 Calories section. If you weigh more than 21 st 6 lb (137 kg), you will need additional calories as described in the chart above.

Get a pen and draw a thick line over the dotted line to the right of your calorie selection. Everything to the left is your ideal daily food intake.

your questions

I really love fruit, so it's been tough for me to eat it only once a day over the past 4 weeks. Once I reach my goal, may I add more fruit servings to my food plan?

You can eat more fruit as long as you substitute another food in its place. The best strategy is to substitute two Treats and Cravings for every extra serving of fruit. But first, try splitting the one serving in half so that you can eat fruit twice a day.

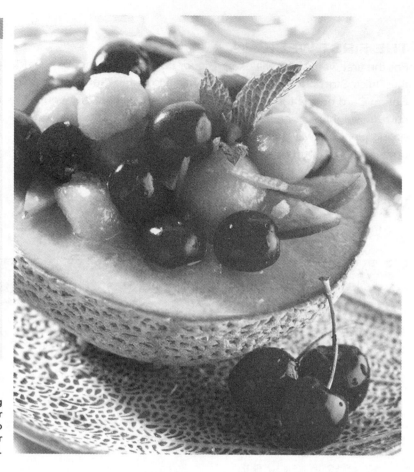

Limiting yourself to just one serving of fruit a day will lower your consumption of simple sugars, keep your insulin levels steady and lower your calorie intake.

treats and cravings

No food is a bad food. True, some foods are a lot better for you than others, but I don't put any food on the 'do not ever eat' list. That just sets you up for bingeing – as soon as you tell yourself that you are not allowed to eat something ever again, you want that food all the more. The foods in my Treats and Cravings category may not be the best foods for your health, but if you love them, you have to find a way to work them into your Eat Fat to Get Fit programme.

Consult the Food List on page 214. I list some of the most highly craved foods, from ice cream to french fries, how much of them you can have, and how many boxes to cross off on your Eating Cards. As long as you limit yourself to a small serving size, you can eat whatever food you want. If you want to go wild on a large-size dessert, make the bulk of your main meal healthy, low-calorie greens. You must still follow your Eating Card System, and once you cross off all the boxes, you've finished eating for the day.

To prevent yourself from overdoing it with Treats and Cravings, heed the following advice.

Tips for Resisting Cravings
Wait 10 minutes before indulging. Most cravings last only about 10 minutes and then subside. Cravings often are your body's cries for water and oxygen. So during those 10 minutes, drink a glass of water with lemon and take a few deep breaths. By giving your body these things, you can easily get through a craving. You might even want to change activities to clear your mind. Go for a walk or take a shower.

Brush your teeth and tongue. This will get the taste of food out of your mouth and ruin the idea of eating something indulgent like fudge. (Chocolate and toothpaste simply don't go together.) Food is less tempting when your mouth feels clean.

Never skip a meal. If you skip a meal, you will feel ravenous and out of control. Be sure to enjoy every one of your meals.

snack happy

Little extras such as chocolates and sweets can help you lose weight by:

- Preventing bingeing
- Making you happy
- Preventing you from feeling deprived

'Your body needs water for everything from maintaining blood volume to skin health to toxin release. Without it, your energy level plummets, you get headaches and you simply don't feel like exercising.'

water

Although not a food category, water is an essential component of my Eat Fat to Get Fit programme. The typical person needs eight 8-fl oz (240-ml) glasses of water a day just for basic maintenance. Most people drink only four to five glasses.

Your body needs water for everything from maintaining blood volume to skin health to toxin release. Without it, your energy level plummets, you get headaches and you simply don't feel like exercising. Even mild dehydration (if you feel thirsty, you're already dehydrated) can make you feel tired. That's because the electrical and chemical signals in your brain ride on water. Dehydration also lowers your blood volume, making your heart pump harder to move blood throughout your body. That tires you out, too. Feeling tired means you won't have the energy to exercise, and you'll burn fewer calories.

Water As Food
Water takes up room in your stomach, making you feel full. That means you eat less and feel less hungry. At parties, keep a glass of water in your hand and sip it instead of grabbing a high-calorie mixed drink or reaching for the snacks. And research shows that many people mistake thirst for hunger, so it's not a bad idea to gulp a glass of water every time you feel a craving, and then decide if you truly *need* to eat.

Of all the ways you can get fluid into your body, drinking water is the best because it has no calories. Zero. If you don't stick to water, your liquid calories can really add up. For example, just 4 fl oz (120 ml) of fruit juice contains 45 to 80 calories. And most people drink a lot more than 4 fl oz (120 ml). A typical bottle of fruit juice drink can contain 150 calories or more. The cafe latte from your favourite coffeeshop chain can contain a whopping 320 calories. And that litre of cola at the cinema contains more than 400 calories. 'Diet' drinks are no better. Most of them contain caffeine, which boosts insulin secretion, making you feel hungry. Caffeine is also a diuretic, which will increase your urine output and make you feel thirsty. And even caffeine-free diet drinks contain high amounts of sodium, which will make you retain water and make you feel bloated and fat.

The worst drink is alcohol; don't drink it at all if you want to lose weight and feel great. It is very high in calories – almost equal to fat calories. If you do have an alcoholic drink, cross off 2 Fat boxes on your Eating Cards, as specified for each amount. Drinking beer will require that you also cross off 1 Complex Carbohydrate box.

tips for switching

It's easy to tell you all the things that are wrong with fruit drinks, coffee, diet drinks and alcohol. It's another thing for you to just switch to drinking water all the time. Here are some tips to help you make the transition.

- Create a concoction. If you don't like the taste of plain water, jazz it up. Try a sparkling water such as Perrier. Pour it into a glass and add some taste with a squeeze of juice from a lemon, lime, orange, or all three.

- Limit yourself to two or fewer caffeinated drinks a day. I'm not going to make you give up your caffeine fix. But if you're the type of person who drinks diet fizzy drinks from the moment you roll out of bed until the end of the workday, you need to cut back to only two of these drinks a day.

- Make smarter choices. You can continue to have those wonderfully delicious coffee drinks if you will make a few simple switches. First, opt for cappuccino. Because they are made with more bubbles, cappuccinos naturally contain fewer calories than lattes and other coffee drinks. Also, order your cappuccino with skimmed milk, which will bring your count down to only about 80 calories. As for fruit juices, choose lower-calorie tomato juice and cranberry juice (with no sugar added). Mix higher-calorie juices with water to lower the calorie count even further.

eating fit at restaurants

Eating out is one of the scariest prospects that dieters face. There are so many tempting sights and smells. But you can eat out – in fact, you can eat anywhere – and still stick to your Eat Fat to Get Fit plan. Just follow these tips:

- Think of your Eating Card the same way you do your credit card: never leave home without it.
- Know that you are the one who is paying the bill and that you are the one in charge. Look at the menu, ask questions and make substitutions when necessary.
- Ask for dressings and sauces to be served on the side.
- When your plate arrives, portion your food before you start to eat. Leave the rest.
- Use extra-virgin olive oil instead of butter.
- Don't forget to eyeball your portion sizes; most restaurants are notorious for overfeeding people.
- Avoid all-you-can-eat buffets.
- Have a salad or vegetables instead of french fries.
- Don't eat from anyone else's plate; that counts, too.

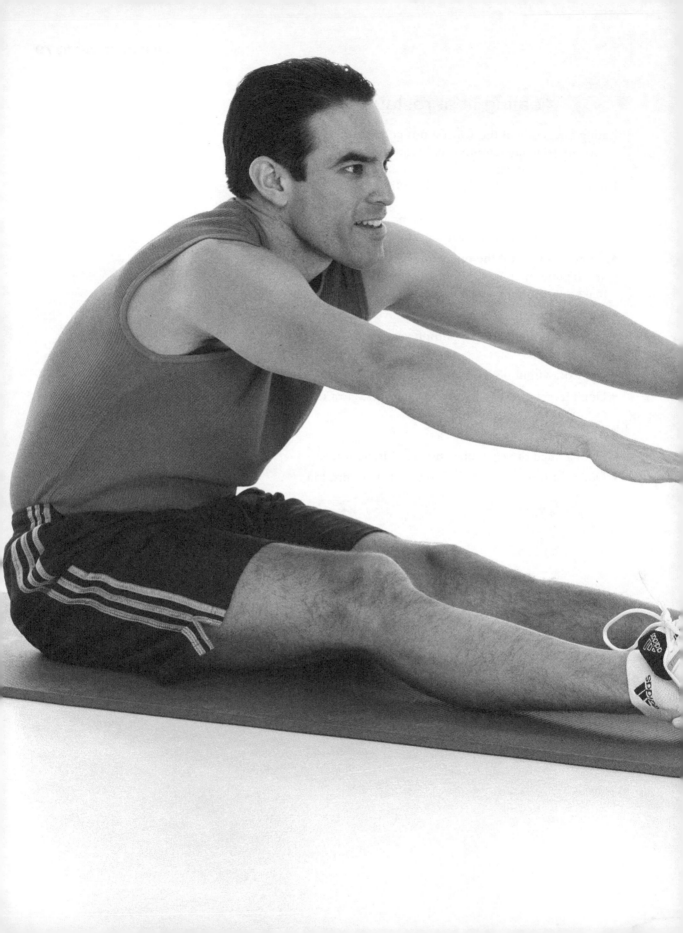

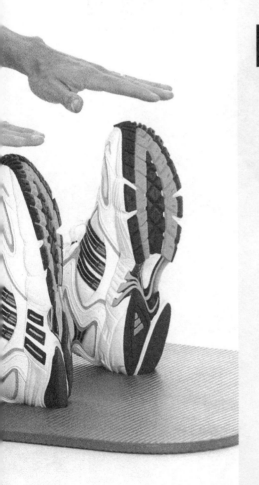

3
The Programme

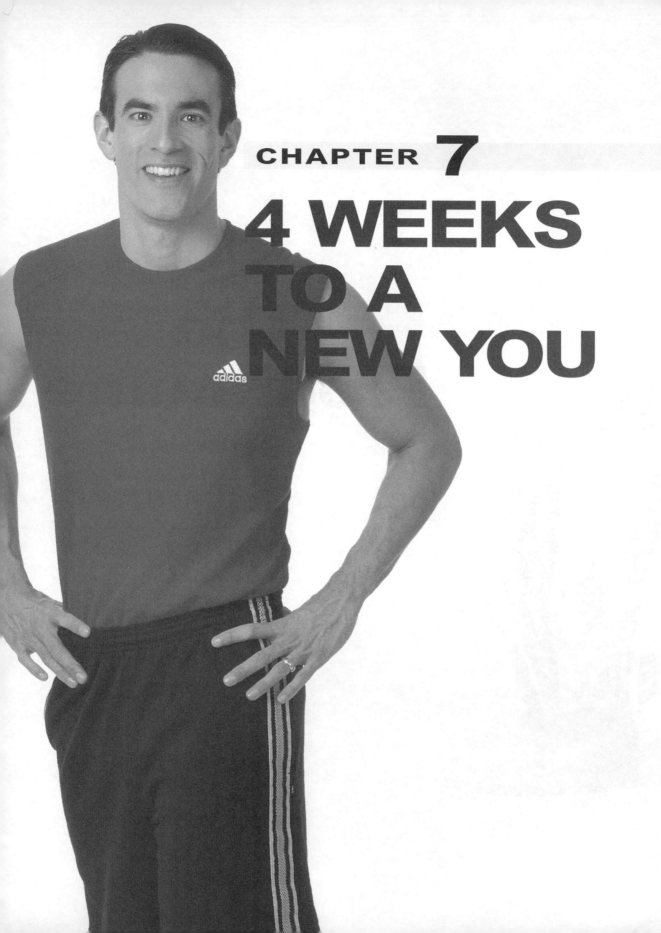

CHAPTER **7**

4 WEEKS TO A NEW YOU

putting jorge's plan into action

'Writing your goals and thoughts will personalize your programme.'

It's time for us to start training together every day for the next 4 weeks. Everything you will need to achieve success will be right here. Each day of this 28-day programme, you will take three simple steps:

1 Read Your Wake-Up Talk found on the first page of each day of the programme. These talks will keep you energized and motivated during the next 4 weeks and will help you get fit from the inside out. Never skip them; they're important.

2 Perform the two Today's Moves training exercises included within each day. To do these exercises correctly, use a weight heavy enough that you feel fatigued by the 12th repetition. Switch back and forth between the two exercises for a total of four times for each exercise without resting. Make sure you warm up before you strength train, and do the three cooldown stretches in 'Warmup and Cooldown'. Use your daily exercise log to help you check off each set you perform. As the 12 repetitions get easier, move up to a heavier weight so that you continue to make rapid progress. Not all of the exercises require a dumbbell, so you can leave the 'lb/kg' column blank for those exercises. As you progress through the programme, you may want to add wrist or ankle weights to them. In that case, use the 'lb/kg' column to record that weight. The log isn't helpful if you don't use it, so keep a pen handy!

3 Use the Eating Card System found starting on page 234. Photocopy the cards you need

your questions

What if I stop seeing progress during the 8 Minutes in the Morning programme?

If this happens to you, just focus on what you want immediately. Don't waste time focusing on the problem. Ask yourself if you are following the Eating Card System precisely and doing your 8 Minutes in the Morning workouts consistently. If so, then you may need to 'jump-start' your success by doing two things. First, follow the Quick Start portion of the Eating Card for the next 7 days. At the same time, if you are not feeling fatigued by the 12th repetition of your morning strength-training exercises, start using heavier dumbbells.

warming up
and cooling down

Start your session with a short warmup to increase the temperature of your body and your joints. When your joints are cold, the fluid inside is thicker, making your joints feel stiff. Save stretching until after strength training to avoid muscle pulls and injuries. As with the rest of the 8 Minutes in the Morning programme, your warm-up is simple.

warmup

Jog in place. Make sure to move both your arms and legs. How fast should you move? On a scale from 1 to 10, aim for a 4 or 5, which is 40 to 50 per cent of your maximum heart rate.

cooldown

Cool down with a quick full-body stretching routine (see photographs). This will increase your range of motion so you stay flexible and avoid injuries.

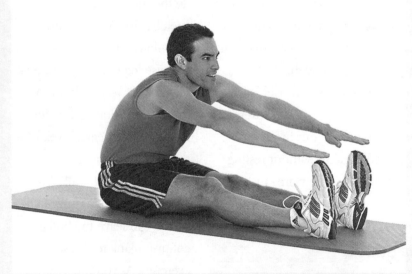

Hurdler's Stretch Sit on a mat on the floor with your legs extended in front of you. Keeping your back flat, gently bend forward from the hips and reach as far as you can towards your toes. If possible, pull your toes back slightly towards your upper body. Hold for 10 seconds to 1 minute.

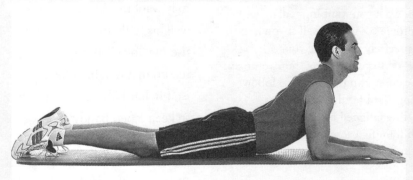

Cobra Stretch Lie on a mat on your belly with your palms flat on the ground next to your shoulders and your legs just slightly less than shoulder-width apart. Your feet should be resting on their tops. Lift your upper body up off the ground, inhaling through your nose as you rise. Press your hips into the floor and curve your upper body backwards, looking up. Hold for 10 seconds to 1 minute.

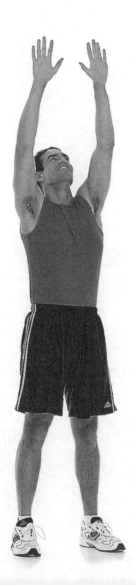

for the week, and always carry them with you to help you keep track of your portions (see page 74 to review how to use the Eating Cards). Be sure to read the food tip each day, which will help you Eat Fat to Get Fit. Use the journal space to write down your thoughts and breakthroughs while living this programme. This book is meant to be interactive and cannot be finalized without your input. Writing your goals and thoughts will personalize your programme. Keeping a journal will teach you more about you. When you add the information that is uniquely yours, this book will be the most important book you own.

get ready to go

I recommend that you start the programme on a Monday. That will allow you to take every Sunday off from exercising (but keep using your Eating Cards), giving you an opportunity to rest, weigh in and prepare for the next week. If you have completed all the tasks on the list below, then you're ready to get started on your first day of the programme.

• Have your dumbbells, a chair, and a mat or towel ready for action.

• Photocopy the master Eating Cards from page 235.

• Have your 'before' photo taken and taped on page 39. If you have not yet taken it, do it today! This will serve as one of the best ways to accurately assess your progress.

• Fill out the Success Contract on page 43; if you haven't finished it, do that now! This will help you stay focused and committed to your goal. Let's go!

Sky-Reaching Pose Stand tall and reach with both hands towards the sky. Reach as high as you comfortably can. Feel the stretch lengthening your spine, bringing more range of motion to your joints. Breathe deeply through your nose. Hold for 10 seconds to 1 minute.

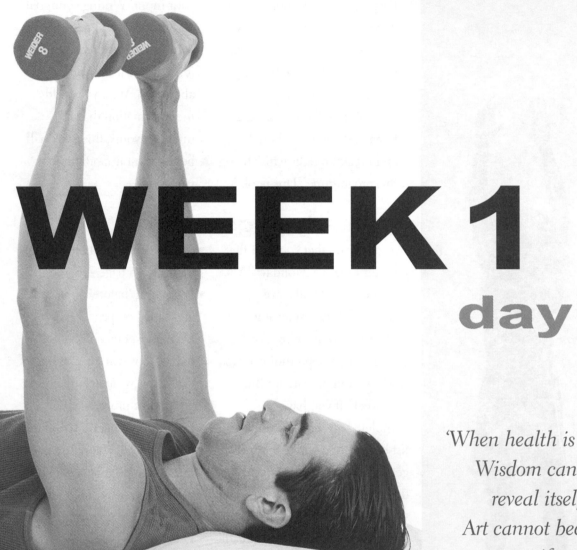

WEEK 1
day 1

'When health is absent
Wisdom cannot
reveal itself,
Art cannot become
manifest,
Strength cannot
be exerted,
Wealth is useless, and
Reason is powerless.'

Herophilus, 300 BC

your wake-up talk

Have you ever known someone who was so passionate and emotional that nothing could stand in the way? Throughout history, people such as Henry Ford, the Wright brothers, Bill Gates, Nelson Mandela and Mother Teresa all had a passion so strong that no matter the obstacles, they made their dreams come true. What was their secret to staying so driven? How did they ignite their passion every day? They each had a very clear plan, a mental blueprint, that guided them successfully to their targets.

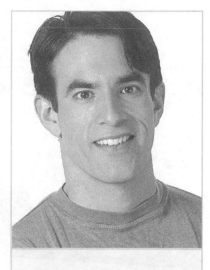

'Having a mental blueprint is critical to your success.'

know what you want

You need a similar passion to build your dream body. Having a mental blueprint is critical to your success. With a clear target, you have the most powerful advantage to making your dream body a reality. Imagine trying to build a house without a blueprint or travelling to a new place without a road map.

Start by designing your ultimate body. Grab a pen and write down what your new body will look like in 'What Is My Specific Goal?' Will you have a defined face, sculpted arms, lean legs, a flat stomach? *Imagine the ideal you and describe what you see.* When you finish, start your 8 Minutes in the Morning workout.

what is my specific goal?

_____

_____

_____

_____

_____

_____

_____

_____

_____

_____

today's moves
chest and
back

A chest dumbbell press

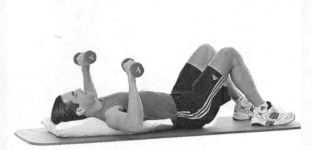 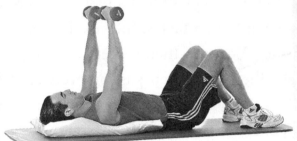

1 Lie on a mat on your back with your knees bent and your feet flat on the floor. You may place one or more pillows under your back and head for support. Holding a dumbbell in each hand, bring your elbows in line with your shoulders, making a right-angle between your upper arm and your side.

2 Exhale as you slowly extend your arms and press the dumbbells towards the ceiling. Keep your elbows slightly bent. Hold for 1 second. Inhale as you return to the starting point.

eat fat to get fit

Dehydration can slow your metabolism by 3 per cent. If you weigh 10 st 10 lb (68 kg), that amounts to 45 fewer calories burned each day. That's the amount in 2 teaspoons of sugar. Even though that doesn't sound like a lot, think in the long term.

That 45 calories a day can prevent your body from burning 5 lb (2.25 kg) of fat a year. It adds up! Few people drink as much water as they should. If you feel thirsty, you are already dehydrated, so don't rely on your body to tell you when to drink.

Instead, drink water on a regular basis. Keep a large water bottle at your desk and take generous sips frequently. Drink a tall glass of water before and after your 8 Minutes in the Morning workout, at your lunch break, and before dinner.

exercise sequence

Warmup
Start your session with a short warmup: jog in place (see page 84).

Training exercises
Do one set of 12 repetitions from exercise A, followed immediately with the same from exercise B. Repeat this cycle for a total of four sets of each exercise, checking them off on your log as you go (see box left).

Cooldown
Finish your session with these three cooldown stretches (see pages 84–5 for full instructions).

Sky-reaching pose: hold for 10 seconds to 1 minute

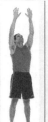

Hurdler's stretch: hold for 10 seconds to 1 minute

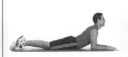

Cobra stretch: hold for 10 seconds to 1 minute

B back two-arm row

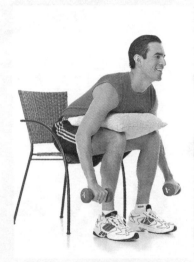

1 Sit in a sturdy chair and grasp a dumbbell in each hand. You may put a pillow on your lap for support. Lean forward and extend your arms straight down, being sure to keep your elbows slightly bent.

2 Exhale as you slowly bend your elbows and bring them towards the ceiling. Once the dumbbells reach the top of your thighs, hold for 1 second. Inhale as you slowly lower the dumbbells to the starting point.

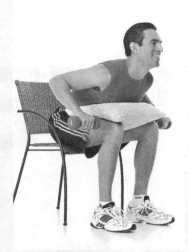

today's journal _____   _____

_____   _____

_____   _____

_____   _____

_____   _____

_____   _____

_____   _____

_____   _____

WEEK 1
day 2

'The future
depends on
what we do in
the present.'

Mahatma Gandhi
Indian nationalist leader

your wake-up talk

Remember the character Ebenezer Scrooge in Charles Dickens's A *Christmas Carol*? Scrooge was a selfish and mean old man who changed his behaviour literally overnight, waking the next day ready for a better life after three ghosts visited him and pointed out his evil ways. When he looked at his life as an observer rather than as a participant, he felt so bad about his actions that he said, 'Enough!'

get dissatisfied now!

Have you ever been so angry, sad or disappointed at something you had been doing that you finally said, 'Enough! I will no longer do this!' That is what you must do right now. Make dissatisfaction work for you. It is one of the most valuable motivational tools you can use to ignite that spark inside you. What has being fat and unfit cost you in your career, your intimate relationships, your family relationships and your personal happiness? Be honest with yourself. Dissatisfaction can provide you with the genesis of your success. Take a few minutes right now to capture your feelings about what inactivity and overeating have cost you. Pick up your pen and write them down in 'What Pain Has Being Unfit Caused Me?'

'Make dissatisfaction work for you.'

what pain has being unfit caused me?

_____
_____
_____
_____
_____
_____
_____
_____
_____
_____
_____

today's moves
shoulders and
abdominals

A shoulders lateral raise

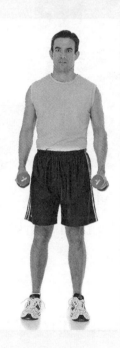

1 Stand with your feet shoulder-width apart, your back straight and your abs tight. Hold a dumbbell in each hand at your sides with your arms straight and your elbows slightly bent.

2 Exhale as you slowly lift the dumbbells out to the side until they are slightly above shoulder level and your palms are facing the floor. Hold for 1 second. Inhale as you lower your arms to the starting point.

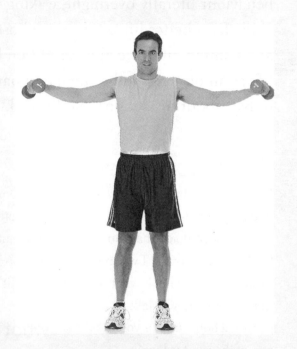

eat fat to get fit

A lot of people overeat not because they are hungry but simply because the food is there. To help yourself stick to the portions that correspond to your calorie selection, dish the correct portions onto your plate and leave the rest of the food in the kitchen. Don't bring it to the table where you might be tempted to indulge in seconds.

Do the same with your snacks. Buy your 'Treats and Cravings' items such as crisps and sweets in small packs or individual servings so that you won't be tempted to down a family-size pack while you watch TV or talk on the phone. And never *ever* eat ice cream straight from the container.

exercise sequence

Warmup
Start your session with a short warmup: jog in place (see page 84).

Training exercises
Do one set of 12 repetitions from exercise A, followed immediately with the same from exercise B. Repeat this cycle for a total of four sets of each exercise, checking them off on your log as you go (see box left).

Cooldown
Finish your session with these three cooldown stretches (see pages 84–5 for full instructions).

Sky-reaching pose: hold for 10 seconds to 1 minute

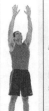

Hurdler's stretch: hold for 10 seconds to 1 minute

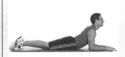

Cobra stretch: hold for 10 seconds to 1 minute

B abdominals crunch

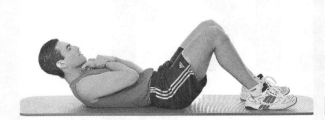
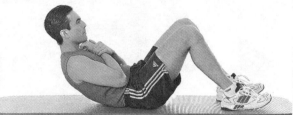

1 Lie on a mat on your back with your knees bent and your feet flat on the floor. Make a fist with one hand and place it between your chin and collarbone. With your other hand, grasp your wrist. This will prevent you from leading with your head and straining your neck.

2 Without moving your lower body, exhale and slowly curl your upper torso until your shoulder blades are off the ground. Hold for 1 second. Inhale as you slowly lower yourself to the starting position.

today's journal_____ _____

_____ _____
_____ _____
_____ _____
_____ _____
_____ _____
_____ _____
_____ _____
_____ _____

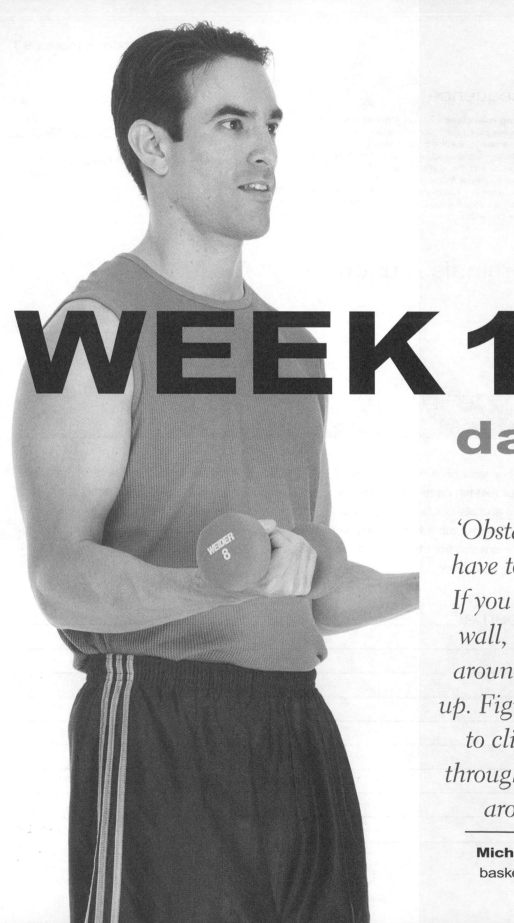

WEEK 1

day 3

'Obstacles don't have to stop you. If you run into a wall, don't turn around and give up. Figure out how to climb it, go through it or work around it.'

Michael Jordan
basketball player

your wake-up talk

For many years, Randy Leamer had unsuccessfully tried to lose weight. But then one day, he became very motivated. Within a year, he lost more than 7 st 5 lb (46 kg). How did he do it? Where did he find that motivation?

know what you will gain

Randy had what I call a Passion Reason (PR). His 5-year-old daughter was in serious need of a kidney transplant, and Randy was the only match. But he was so obese that doctors didn't want to perform the surgery; it was too risky. So without hesitation, Randy started eating properly and exercising daily. For the next 11 months, he never complained and never missed a workout. Once he lost the weight, he was able to donate his kidney and save his daughter's life. He has kept the weight off ever since.

You must find your own Passion Reasons by creating a Power List. Write down the three most important things in your life – your partner, your family, financial freedom, your spirituality, and so on.

Then ask yourself what you will gain by losing weight. Your answer to that question will help you create Passion Reasons (two for each item on your list). If you put your partner on your Power List, you might answer 'more romance and better sex'. If it's financial independence, you might write down 'more energy to start home business'.

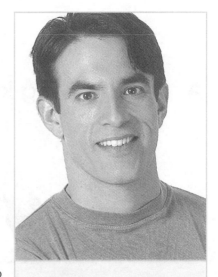

'Ask yourself what you will gain by losing weight.'

Review your Passion Reasons every day!

my power list
1 _____
pr_____
pr_____
2 _____
pr_____
pr_____
3 _____
pr_____
pr_____

today's moves
triceps and
biceps

A triceps lying kickback

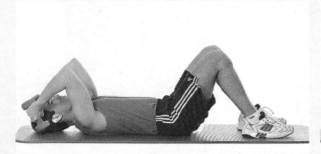 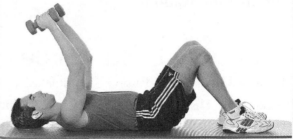

1 Lie on a mat on your back with a dumbbell in each hand by your ears and your elbows pointing up.

2 Exhale as you slowly extend your arms and raise the dumbbells towards the ceiling. Straighten your arms but keep your elbows slightly bent. Hold for 1 second. Inhale as you lower the dumbbells to the starting point.

eat fat to get fit

Even though fruit juice is loaded with vitamins and antioxidants that can improve your health, most types are also loaded with calories. One 10-fl oz (300-ml) bottle can contain 150 calories.

If you love juice and want its nutritional goodness but don't want the calories, dilute it. Fill your glass halfway with sparkling water and the rest of the way with your fruit juice. That will cut the calorie count in half without sacrificing the taste. You can also add sparkling water to wine, tomato juice and even fizzy drinks. Over time, you can wean yourself from caloric drinks altogether by increasing the amount of sparkling water. Eventually, you'll be drinking sparkling water with only a hint of juice for taste.

exercise sequence

Warmup
Start your session with a short warmup: jog in place (see page 84).

Training exercises
Do one set of 12 repetitions from exercise A, followed immediately with the same from exercise B. Repeat this cycle for a total of four sets of each exercise, checking them off on your log as you go (see box left).

Cooldown
Finish your session with these three cooldown stretches (see pages 84–5 for full instructions).

Sky-reaching pose: hold for 10 seconds to 1 minute

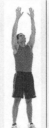

Hurdler's stretch: hold for 10 seconds to 1 minute

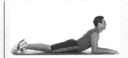

Cobra stretch: hold for 10 seconds to 1 minute

B biceps standing curl

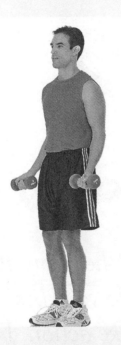

1 Stand with your feet shoulder-width apart and your arms extended by your sides. Hold a dumbbell in each hand, palms facing forward.

2 Exhale as you simultaneously curl both arms to just past 90 degrees, bringing your palms towards your biceps. Keep your elbows close to your sides and concentrate on moving only from your elbow joints, not from your shoulders. Hold for 1 second. Inhale as you return to the starting point.

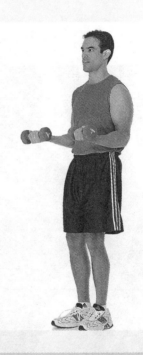

today's journal _____ _____

_____ _____
_____ _____
_____ _____
_____ _____
_____ _____
_____ _____
_____ _____

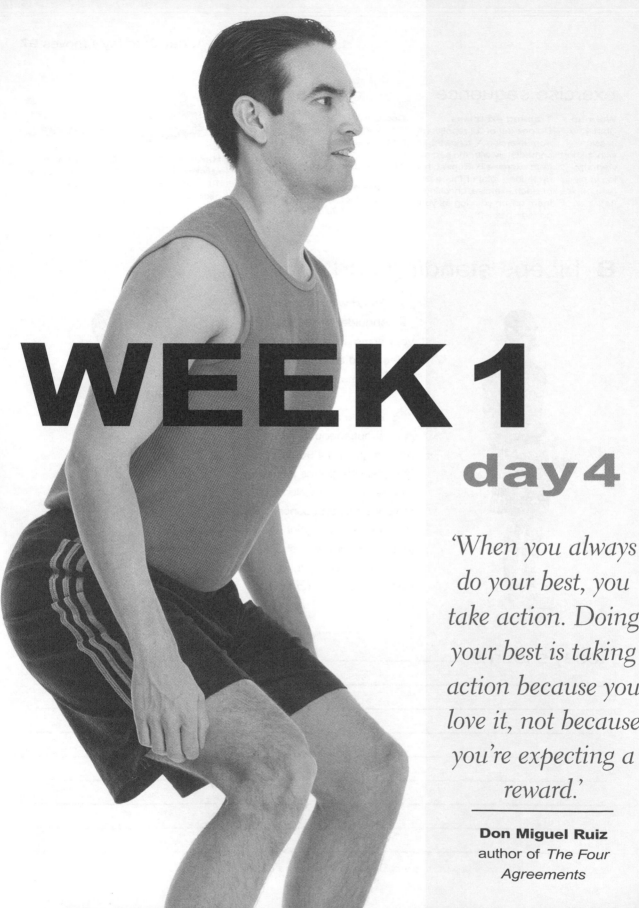

WEEK 1
day 4

'When you always do your best, you take action. Doing your best is taking action because you love it, not because you're expecting a reward.'

Don Miguel Ruiz
author of *The Four Agreements*

your wake-up talk

Being able to vividly see your ideal body is a critical step in achieving that body. Think about any item in the physical world: a car, a computer, or a dress. It did not get here by accident. It's here because someone saw a very clear mental image of what they wanted to create before it existed. That is what I want you to experience right now. I want you to see the body that you will have in the future. Practising visualization (see 'Visualization Exercise') each morning will allow you to see and feel the new you that is emerging.

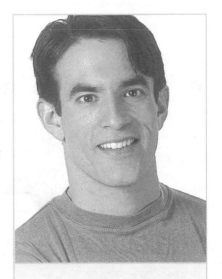

'Visualize the body that you will have in the future.'

visualization exercise

1 Close your eyes; take a few deep, relaxing breaths through your nose; and see yourself through the lens of a camera.

Look at yourself with the body you want to have. How is your posture? What are you wearing?

If you are seeing a black-and-white picture of yourself, add colour. Put a big smile on your face.

2 With your eyes still closed, see yourself through the lens of a video camera. This means that you can stretch, walk, dance, run, laugh and interact with the environment you are in. See the body you want to have.

3 Jump into the body that you want. You can now see things through your own eyes. Look at the tone in your arms and legs; it is yours to enjoy.

today's moves
hamstrings and
quadriceps

EXERCISE LOG					
exercise	lb/kg	set 1 ✓	set 2 ✓	set 3 ✓	set 4 ✓
A					
B					

A hamstrings leg lift

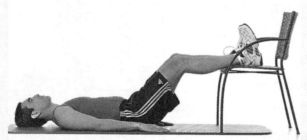 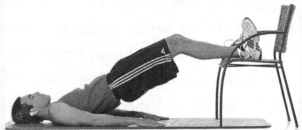

1 Lie on a mat with your palms flat on the floor and your heels on the seat of a sturdy chair.

2 Exhale as you slowly contract the backs of your upper thighs to push your buttocks towards the ceiling. Hold for 1 second. Inhale as you slowly lower your buttocks to the starting point.

eat fat to get fit

Olive oil is one of the more healthy oils to cook with, which is why I recommend it in my Eat Fat to Get Fit eating programme. There are many varieties, and it can be very confusing deciding which one to buy. From pure to extra-virgin, the best one really depends on your taste buds and your budget. Extra-virgin is the most expensive and highest-quality olive oil. Extra-virgin oil must come from the first pressing of the olives: it is extracted gently, without using heat or chemicals and is unrefined, giving the oil a rich flavour. Virgin olive oil is also cold-pressed and unrefined, with a good flavour. Pure olive oil is extracted from a second or third pressing, using heat, and is then refined; it has a less noticeable olive flavour.

exercise sequence

Warmup
Start your session with a short warmup: jog in place (see page 84).

Training exercises
Do one set of 12 repetitions from exercise A, followed immediately with the same from exercise B. Repeat this cycle for a total of four sets of each exercise, checking them off on your log as you go (see box left).

Cooldown
Finish your session with these three cooldown stretches (see pages 84–5 for full instructions).

Sky-reaching pose: hold for 10 seconds to 1 minute

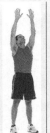

Hurdler's stretch: hold for 10 seconds to 1 minute

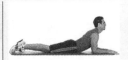

Cobra stretch: hold for 10 seconds to 1 minute

B quadriceps squat

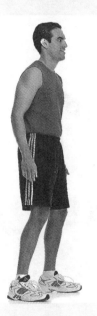

1 Stand with your feet slightly wider than shoulder-width apart and your arms at your sides. Keeping your back straight and your abs tight, exhale as you slowly squat down to about 90 degrees.

2 Push your backside out as if you were sitting into a chair and don't let your knees extend forward past your toes. If you need to, you can rest your hands on your thighs. Hold for 1 second. Inhale as you slowly return to the starting position.

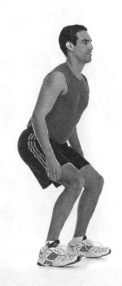

today's journal _____   _____
_____   _____
_____   _____
_____   _____
_____   _____
_____   _____
_____   _____
_____   _____

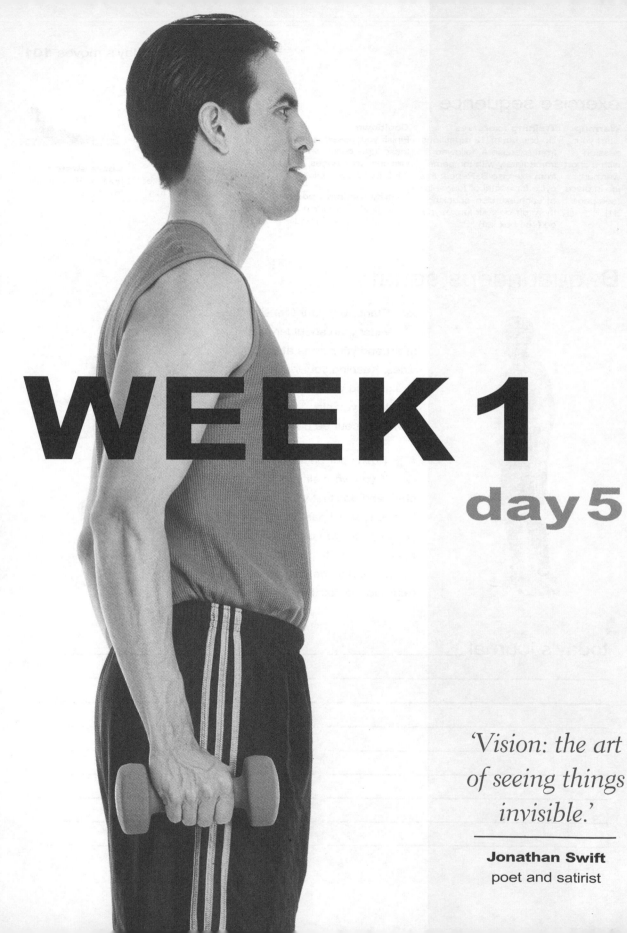

WEEK 1
day 5

'Vision: the art
of seeing things
invisible.'

Jonathan Swift
poet and satirist

your wake-up talk

Do you remember the movie *Forrest Gump*? It is about a man who leads an extraordinary life even though he is 'handicapped'. Forrest is able to make all his dreams come true because of the way his mother taught him to see the world. She helped him master the ultimate environment: his internal one.

create the ultimate environment

She explained things in a way that made Forrest ask what I call Result-Driven Questions (RDQs). Instead of asking himself, 'Why am I disabled?', 'What's wrong with my legs?' or 'Why I am I slower than all the other kids?' he asks questions such as, 'Why did God make me so special?', 'Why am I so lucky to have these magic shoes?' or 'How do miracles happen every day?'

By asking Result-Driven Questions, you are actually unable to focus on things that make you depressed or unmotivated. You have no option but to see things in a way that empowers you.

If you ask negatively driven questions such as 'Why can't I lose weight?' or 'What's my problem?' your answers will reveal all of the reasons why you can't lose the weight and will make you feel worse. Using RDQs will give you the power to direct what you see and hear; they direct your emotions towards the results you want. You need to read and think about the RDQs each and every day.

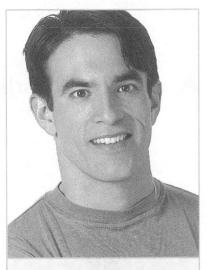

'Read and think about result-driven questions every day.'

result-driven questions

Photocopy these RDQs and place them on your refrigerator, at your desk at work, or on your closet door so that you'll see them often.

1 What joy will I feel when I attain my ultimate body?

2 How incredible will my life become when I am leaner?

3 What extraordinary things will people say to me when I am leaner?

4 How will I see my body transform with the healthy choices I make?

5 What can I do today so that my weight-loss plans run smoothly?

6 How can I continue to create a weight-loss support network?

today's moves
calves and
buttocks

EXERCISE LOG					
exercise	lb/kg	set 1 ✓	set 2 ✓	set 3 ✓	set 4 ✓
A					
B					

A calves standing heel raise

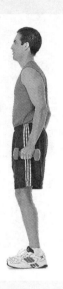

1 Stand with your feet shoulder-width apart. Hold a dumbbell in each hand at your sides with your arms extended but not locked. Keep your chest out, your shoulder blades rolled back and down and your abs tight.

2 Exhale as you slowly lift your heels and rise onto your tiptoes. Hold for 1 second. Inhale as you slowly lower yourself to the starting position.

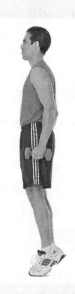

eat fat to get fit

A lot of people tell me that they hardly eat anything, but still can't manage to lose weight. I ask them to think about all of those little calories that most people tend to think of as 'freebies' or don't count as food actually eaten. For many, it's the food they taste as they cook. Those spoonfuls of soup, nibbles of cheese, biscuits or nuts can easily add up to 100 extra calories a day or more. That could amount to an extra 10 lb (4.5 kg) per year! Other overlooked calorie sources include free samples at the supermarket, goodies left on your desk by colleagues and the rest of the food on your child's plate. If you nibble here and there, don't forget to cross off the right boxes on your Eating Cards!

exercise sequence

Warmup
Start your session with a short warmup: jog in place (see page 84).

Training exercises
Do one set of 12 repetitions from exercise A, followed immediately with the same from exercise B. Repeat this cycle for a total of four sets of each exercise, checking them off on your log as you go (see box left).

Cooldown
Finish your session with these three cooldown stretches (see pages 84–5 for full instructions).

Sky-reaching pose: hold for 10 seconds to 1 minute

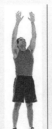

Hurdler's stretch: hold for 10 seconds to 1 minute

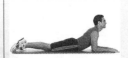

Cobra stretch: hold for 10 seconds to 1 minute

B buttocks kickup

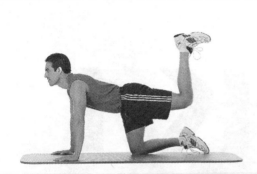

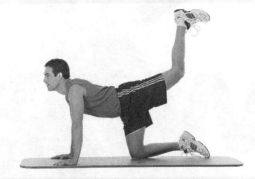

1 Kneel on a mat on all fours with your knees hip-width apart, your hands slightly wider apart than your shoulders and your fingers pointing forward. Keeping your head up, raise your left leg until your thigh is in line with your torso.

2 Bend your knee and exhale as you slowly push your foot towards the ceiling. If this puts too much stress on your back, lower your head so that you are looking down at the mat. Hold for 1 second. Inhale as you slowly lower your leg. Do one set with your left leg, then switch sides.

today's journal _____   _____

_____   _____

_____   _____

_____   _____

_____   _____

_____   _____

_____   _____

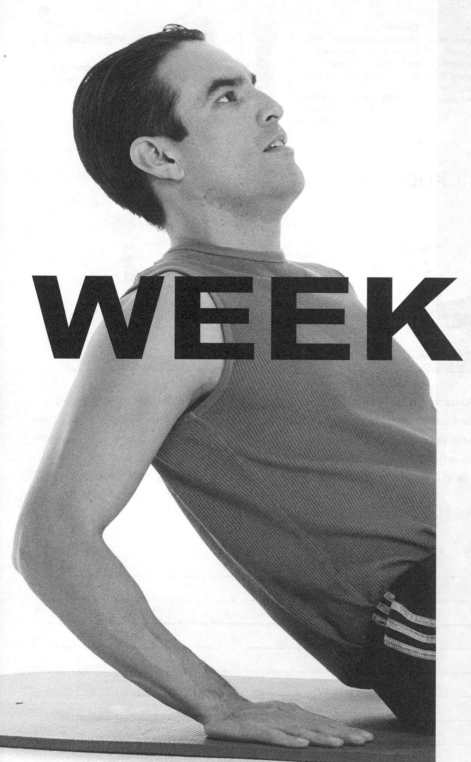

WEEK 1
day 6

'You cannot
depend on your
eyes when your
imagination is
out of focus.'

Mark Twain
writer and satirist

your wake-up talk

How great would it be if you could find an extra 3 to 4 hours each week? How could you use that time to accelerate your success? How much leaner could you get? How much sooner could you achieve your goal?

create more time for you

All of us have what I call a Loser Zone, where most of us spend too much time. You fall into the Loser Zone when you do something that produces no significant improvement in your life. The number one Loser Zone activity is watching television; the average person spends 23 hours a week watching it. Your Loser Zone time might also involve aimlessly chatting on the phone or surfing the Internet.

What are your Loser Zones, and how many hours per day do you spend per Loser Zone activity? If your number is greater than 6 to 8 hours, you have just found some time that could be better spent on creating your best body ever.

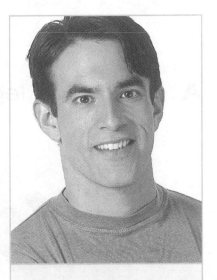

'Identify time that could be better spent on creating your best body ever.'

what are my loser zones?

Loser Zone activity:_____ Hours per day:_____

Loser Zone activity: _____ Hours per day:_____

Loser Zone activity:_____ Hours per day:_____

Total time in Loser Zone:_____ × 7 days =_____

This is how much MORE time you have for yourself per week when you get out of your Loser Zone.

today's moves
inner thigh and
outer thigh

EXERCISE LOG					
exercise	lb/kg	set 1 ✓	set 2 ✓	set 3 ✓	set 4 ✓
A					
B					

A inner thigh leg raise

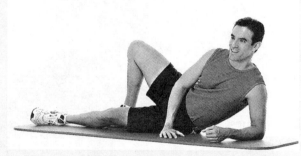 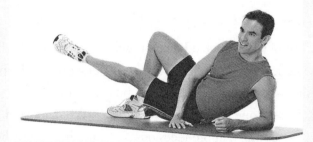

1 Lie on a mat on your left side with your left elbow and forearm supporting your upper body and your left leg extended. Bend your right knee and place your right foot behind your left leg for balance.

2 Keeping your left leg straight, exhale as you slowly lift your left foot as high as you can. Hold for 1 second. Inhale as you lower your foot to the starting position. Do one set with your left leg, then switch sides.

eat fat to get fit

The next time you're in the mood for pizza, order it without cheese. Cheese accounts for most of the calories in the pizza, and it contains lots of unhealthy and fattening saturated fat. If you make your own pizza, use cheese substitutes made from soya, or use no cheese at all. I promise that you will eventually grow to prefer your pizza this way; I know I have. Now after I eat pizza, I feel healthy rather than bloated and sleepy. If you crave a hint of cheese, sprinkle a small amount of Parmesan cheese on top for the flavour without the bad fat and calories.

exercise sequence

Warmup
Start your session with a short warmup: jog in place (see page 84).

Training exercises
Do one set of 12 repetitions from exercise A, followed immediately with the same from exercise B. Repeat this cycle for a total of four sets of each exercise, checking them off on your log as you go (see box left).

Cooldown
Finish your session with these three cooldown stretches (see pages 84–5 for full instructions).

Sky-reaching pose: hold for 10 seconds to 1 minute

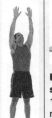

Hurdler's stretch: hold for 10 seconds to 1 minute

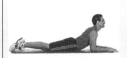

Cobra stretch: hold for 10 seconds to 1 minute

B outer thigh doggie

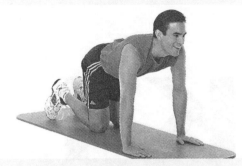

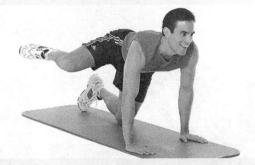

1 Kneel on a mat on all fours with your knees hip-width apart, your hands placed slightly wider than your shoulders and your fingers pointing forward. Keep your back straight and your head up.

2 Keeping your leg bent at a 90-degree angle, exhale as you raise your right leg out to the side. Hold for 1 second. Inhale as you slowly lower your leg back to the starting point. Do one set with your right leg, then switch sides.

today's journal _____

_____
_____
_____
_____
_____
_____
_____
_____
_____

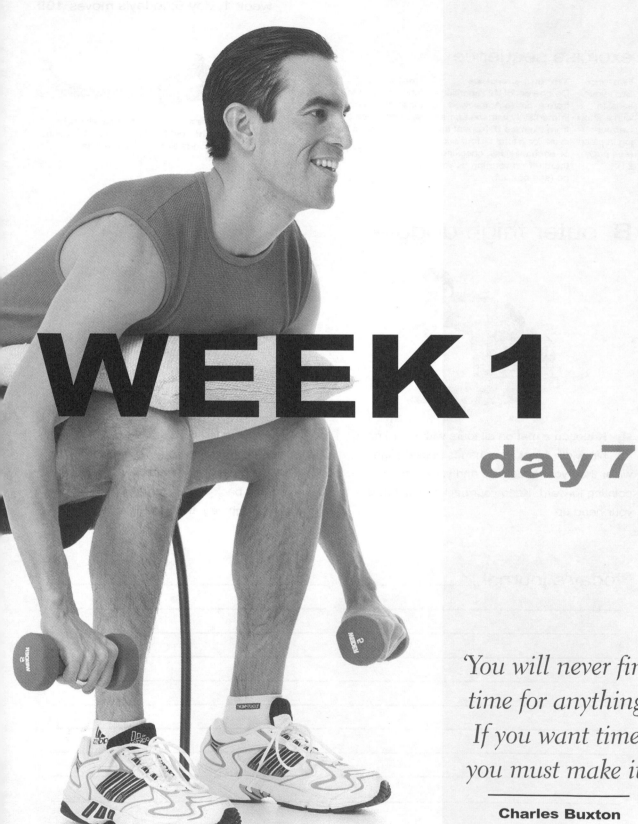

WEEK 1
day 7

'You will never find
time for anything.
If you want time,
you must make it.'

Charles Buxton
writer

your wake-up talk

When you look through your old photo albums, do you feel the emotions captured in the photos? Imagine a special birthday, wedding or graduation photo. Can you put yourself in that moment and feel it again? Photographs have a certain magical power for us; they can move us to feel a certain way almost instantly.

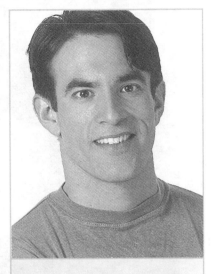

create a power collage

Have you ever seen someone in great shape and thought, 'I want to look like that', then found yourself doing your next set of exercises with more excitement and motivation? You need to surround yourself with motivating images.

I want you to use your time on Sunday of each week to create a power collage. Flip through three or four magazines and select five or more photos of people who are healthy and fit that inspire you. Cut them out and paste them onto poster board. Put your power collage in a place where you will see it

'You need to surround yourself with motivating images.'

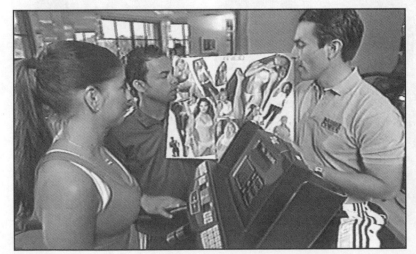

throughout the day and use these images to emotionally fuel your workouts.

This is your day off, so take some extra time for yourself. Go for a powerwalk, get some fresh air and motivate yourself for next week.

Assemble inspiring images on a poster board to form your own power collage.

8 minute marvel Stephanie lost 2 st 4 lb (15 kg)!

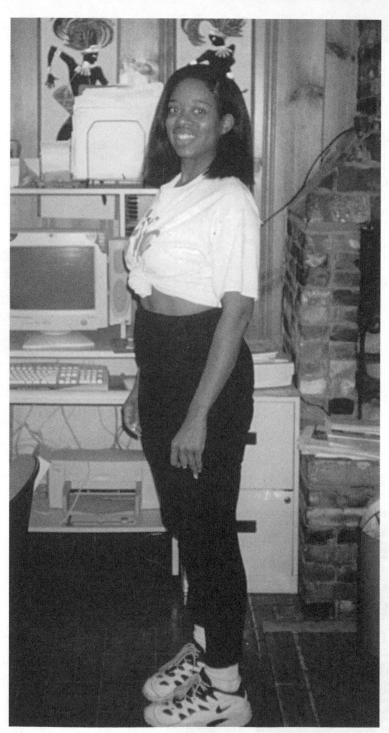

A single mother of two, I've had an extremely difficult time losing weight in the past. After 2 years, I still didn't fit into my pre-pregnancy clothes. I spent months eating low-fat foods and doing 60 minutes of high-impact aerobics every day, but got nowhere. But everything changed when I started the 8 Minutes in the Morning programme.

'My body is now lean, and I have more energy than ever before.'

With the 8 Minutes in the Morning programme guiding me, I always had the tools to accomplish my goals. This programme has changed my life! My friends, family and colleagues always compliment me on my appearance.

Stephanie Donald
Production Manager

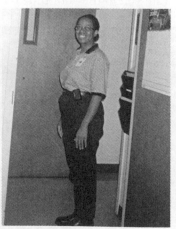

before

eat fat to get fit

Like most people, I like to eat something sweet once in a while. But I don't like to cross off all of those food boxes just for a piece of cake or a couple of biscuits.

So when I'm hankering after a sweet taste, especially just after a meal, I go to my freezer. Not for ice cream, but for frozen seedless grapes.

There's something about a frozen grape that makes it so much more delicious than the room-temperature version, and you can eat 12 of them before you have to cross off your fruit allowance for the day on your Eating Card. And grapes are loaded with healthy phytochemicals that fight off heart disease and cancer.

That's a pretty good way to satisfy your cravings.

IMPORTANT: WEEK 1 UPDATE

It's time to monitor how you are doing and record your first week's progress. This will keep you focused and accountable. Grab a pen and answer the following questions.

1 What is your current weight? Use scales to weigh yourself and also write down your original weight.

_____

2 What have you done well this week? What makes you proud of you?

_____
_____
_____

3 What could you be doing better or improving?

_____
_____
_____
_____
_____

4 What is your game plan for week 2? _____

_____
_____
_____
_____

Interact with

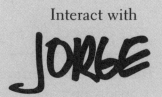

If you would like me to contact you about your progress, send me an e-mail with your answers to this week's update to *weekone@jorgecruise.com*. I will send you a special e-mail with bonus tips on how to make week 2 even more fun and effective.

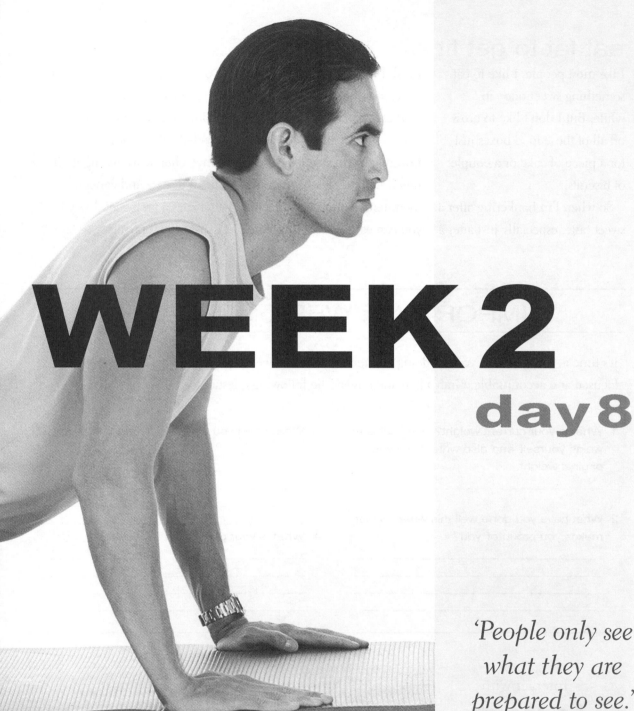

WEEK 2
day 8

'People only see
what they are
prepared to see.'

Ralph Waldo Emerson
philosopher and poet

your wake-up talk

Feeling certain that you will attain your dream body is critical. A feeling of certainty is nothing more than a belief that you will do it. If you know that you will succeed, you will achieve it. How do you strengthen your belief that you will get a lean body? How do you create an unbreakable confidence that your goal will be achieved?

create more certainty now

You need to create 'positive references'. Author Tony Robbins, my friend and mentor, explains the concept this way: think of your belief as a tabletop and the legs of the table as the references that support the tabletop. For example, if you believe that you are smart (tabletop), you have references (legs) that support your belief. Maybe people have told you that you are smart, you have many smart friends and you enjoy doing smart activities such as reading and attending seminars. Similarly, in order to believe that you will become lean, you need legs to support that belief.

Write down at least four references that support the belief that you will lose weight in 'I Will Get Lean'. For example, you might write: 'I have so much to gain with my family', 'I have the support of my family', and 'I am a good role model for my kids'. Review these references daily.

> 'If you know that you will succeed, you will achieve it.'

I will get lean

My four references that support this belief:

1 _____
_____

2 _____
_____

3 _____
_____

4 _____
_____

today's moves
chest and
back

	EXERCISE LOG				
exercise	lb/kg	set 1 ✓	set 2 ✓	set 3 ✓	set 4 ✓
A					
B					

A chest knee pushup

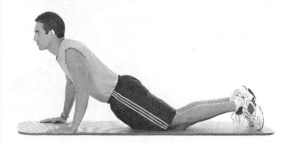

1 Kneel on a mat on all fours with your knees hip-width apart, your hands slightly wider than shoulder-width apart and your fingers pointing forward. Bring your pelvis forward so that your body creates a straight line from your knees to your head.

2 Inhale and lower your chest towards the floor until your elbows are even with your shoulders, keeping your back straight and your abs tight. Exhale and push back up to the starting position, keeping your elbows slightly bent.

eat fat to get fit

As part of the Eat Fat to Get Fit food plan, I recommend eating a lot of vegetables – no less than six servings a day and up to nine servings a day, depending on the calorie selection you are following. Some of my clients have told me that they have trouble fitting this many vegetables into their diets.

My answer to this is to keep cut-up veggies in your refrigerator at home and at work. Use them to satisfy your cravings. Unlike snack foods such as crisps and biscuits, you can eat as many crunchy veggies as you want. Just put a bag of baby carrots, celery sticks or cauliflower florets on your desk and nibble away. The best part is that you don't have to spend a lot of time preparing these veggies. Most supermarkets now sell pre-chopped vegetables so that you can eat them straight from the bag.

exercise sequence

Warmup
Start your session with a short warmup: jog in place (see page 84).

Training exercises
Do one set of 12 repetitions from exercise A, followed immediately with the same from exercise B. Repeat this cycle for a total of four sets of each exercise, checking them off on your log as you go (see box left).

Cooldown
Finish your session with these three cooldown stretches (see pages 84–5 for full instructions).

Sky-reaching pose: hold for 10 seconds to 1 minute

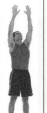

Hurdler's stretch: hold for 10 seconds to 1 minute

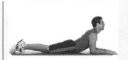

Cobra stretch: hold for 10 seconds to 1 minute

B back bird dog

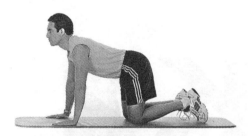

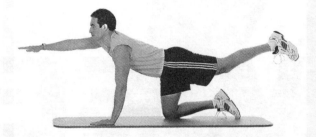

1 Kneel on a mat on all fours with your knees hip-width apart, your hands slightly wider than shoulder-width apart and your fingers pointing forward. Keeping your head up, exhale and simultaneously lift and extend your left arm and your right leg. Keep your back straight and abs tight throughout the move.

2 When your arm and thigh are parallel to the floor, hold for a count of 3. Inhale as you lower them back to the starting position. Repeat with the opposite arm and leg. Continue to switch sides until you have completed one set on each side.

today's journal _____ _____

_____ _____

_____ _____

_____ _____

_____ _____

_____ _____

_____ _____

_____ _____

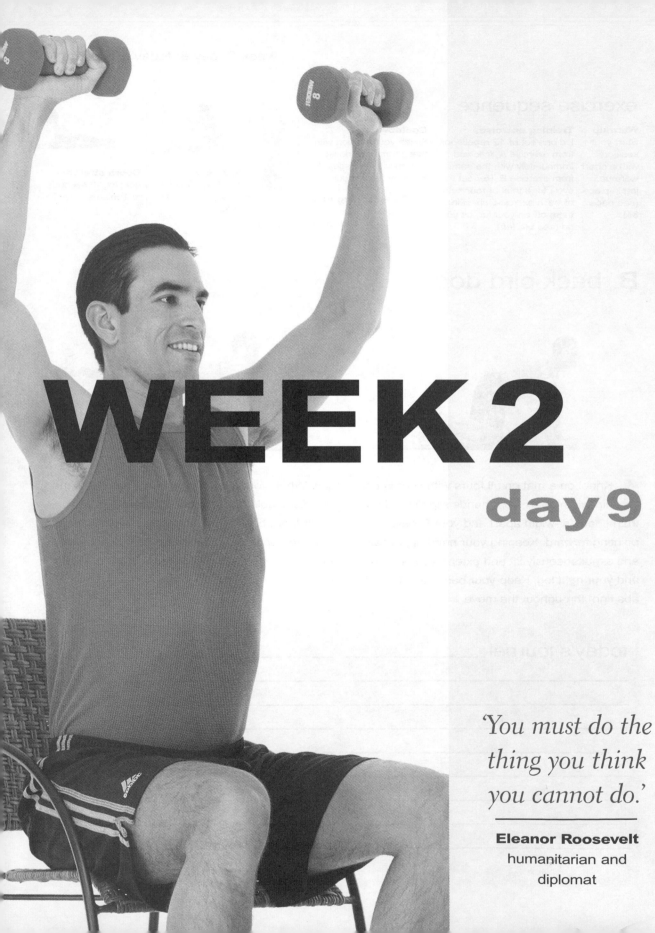

WEEK2
day 9

'You must do the
thing you think
you cannot do.'

Eleanor Roosevelt
humanitarian and
diplomat

your wake-up talk

I have a good friend who once worked at Disneyland at a concession stand. Although it wasn't the highest-paying job, she loved it more than any other job because everywhere else, she was just an employee. At the park, however, she was a cast member. She did not feel as though she was in the concession business, but rather that she was in the entertainment business. She smiled just thinking about her title. This is what I call a Power Label.

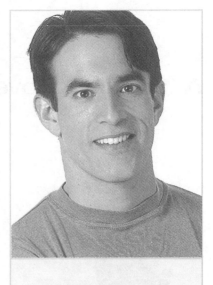

create your power label

For you to achieve your ideal body, you must create a Power Label for yourself that gets you excited about exercising and eating well. Think about it. Too many people unconsciously label themselves in ways that make them feel bad: over the hill, overeater, couch potato, chocoholic, meat-and-potatoes guy or big as a house. The human brain is such a powerful instrument that you will eventually become whatever you label yourself. For example, if you really think that you have a 'sweet tooth', you will always have problems with sweets. But the truth is that nobody really has a sweet tooth. It is just a saying that becomes real only when you take it on. I want you to select a positive Power Label for yourself. Make up something that works for you. The secret is to live it every day!

> 'Select a positive Power Label for yourself.'

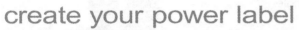

power labels

Sexy Mama	**Strong Power Mum**
Adonis	**Superwoman**
Hot Babe	**Superman**
Athlete	

Choose a Power Label (or make up your own) and write it below. Post it everywhere.

_____

_____

today's moves
shoulders and
abdominals

EXERCISE LOG					
exercise	lb/kg	set 1 ✓	set 2 ✓	set 3 ✓	set 4 ✓
A					
B					

A shoulders overhead press

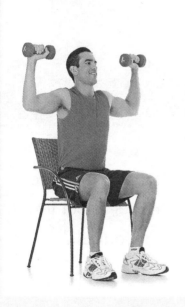

1 Sit on the edge of a sturdy chair with your back straight and your abs tight. Hold a dumbbell in each hand with your hands just above ear level and your palms facing forward. Your upper arms should be parallel to the floor and your elbows bent at a 90-degree angle.

2 Exhale as you slowly straighten your arms and press the dumbbells towards the ceiling, keeping your elbows slightly bent. Hold for 1 second. Inhale as you slowly return to the starting position.

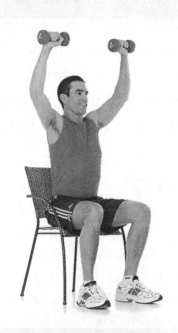

eat fat to get fit

When people tell me that they don't like vegetables, I tell them that they probably haven't cooked them correctly. If you've ever eaten overcooked, mushy brussels sprouts, mangetout or broccoli, you were probably left with a yucky feeling.

I challenge you to give vegetables another chance. This time, take care when you are preparing them. The best ways to cook vegetables are to grill, steam or blanch them; or sauté them in an olive oil spray. Cook them only until they are warm; they should

remain crunchy. Once they become soft, they will lose their taste and texture. Just like pasta, vegetables should always be al dente. You can also punch up the taste by adding lemon juice, garlic or lime juice, none of which will add calories to your meal.

exercise sequence

Warmup
Start your session with a short warmup: jog in place (see page 84).

Training exercises
Do one set of 12 repetitions from exercise A, followed immediately with the same from exercise B. Repeat this cycle for a total of four sets of each exercise, checking them off on your log as you go (see box left).

Cooldown
Finish your session with these three cooldown stretches (see pages 84–5 for full instructions).

Sky-reaching pose: hold for 10 seconds to 1 minute

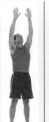

Hurdler's stretch: hold for 10 seconds to 1 minute

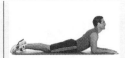

Cobra stretch: hold for 10 seconds to 1 minute

B abdominals lower pull

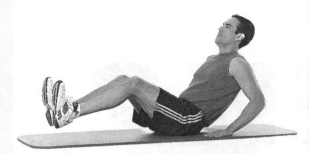

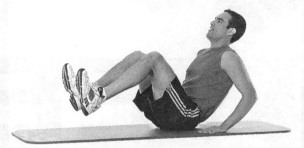

1 Sit on a mat on the floor with your legs slightly bent, your heels just above the floor and your hands behind your buttocks for support. Exhale as you slowly raise your heels and bring your knees towards your torso.

2 When your thighs and abdomen create a 90-degree angle, hold for 1 second. Inhale as you slowly return to the starting position.

today's journal _____ _____

_____ _____

_____ _____

_____ _____

_____ _____

_____ _____

_____ _____

_____ _____

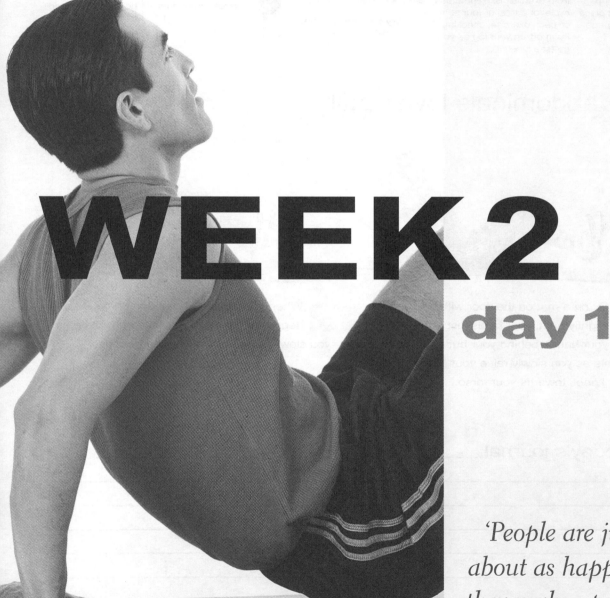

WEEK2

day 10

'People are just about as happy as they make up their minds to be.'

Abraham Lincoln
16th US president

your wake-up talk

Friends of mine have a baby boy named Matthew. I visit my friends once a year, and each time, I am amazed at how much bigger and smarter Matthew has become. But his parents don't notice and see the differences. It's not that they don't care or don't pay attention; it's just that they see him every day. When you are around someone or something every day, you tend to not see the small incremental changes.

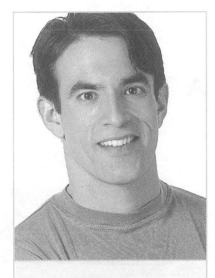

use progress to push forward

It's the same with weight loss; people often lose their motivation because they think that they are not progressing. They think that their efforts are not paying off, which hinders their progress.

One of the most essential things you can do to stay on track and motivated is to record your progress.

I want you to write down the 10 most important things you have learned while participating in the 8 Minutes in the Morning programme. These are things that will help you stay fit for the rest of your life. They can be big things or small things. The secret is to notice that you have changed and then appreciate your progress. Use this list to remind yourself about the person you are now becoming.

'To stay on track and motivated, record your progress.'

10 most important things I have learned

1 _____
2 _____
3 _____
4 _____
5 _____
6 _____
7 _____
8 _____
9 _____
10 _____

today's moves
triceps and
biceps

A triceps dip

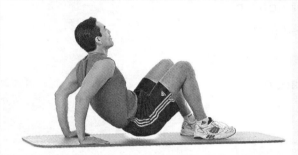 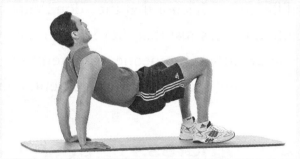

1 Sit on a mat with your legs bent at a 90-degree angle and your hands about 1 ft (30 cm) behind your buttocks for support. Your fingers should face towards you, your arms should be slightly bent and your buttocks should be slightly off the floor. Your buttocks should not touch the floor again until you have finished the exercise.

2 Exhale as you slowly extend your arms, keeping your elbows slightly bent. When your arms are extended, hold for 1 second. Inhale as you lower yourself back to the starting position.

eat fat to get fit

If you've never bought and cooked fish before, give it a try. Salmon, swordfish and tuna all come in steak form, which is great for easy grilling, and difficult to cook incorrectly.

When buying fish, look for cuts that are moist and firm with no dried-out edges. If it has skin, it should be shiny and metallic-looking. When you get the fish home, marinate it. For one of my favourite marinades, combine miso (a soya product) with some balsamic vinegar, olive oil and a touch of soy sauce in a resealable plastic bag, then add the fish. Let it marinate for 45 minutes before grilling or cooking on a hot, ridged stovetop chargrilling pan.

exercise sequence

Warmup
Start your session with a short warmup: jog in place (see page 84).

Training exercises
Do one set of 12 repetitions from exercise A, followed immediately with the same from exercise B. Repeat this cycle for a total of four sets of each exercise, checking them off on your log as you go (see box left).

Cooldown
Finish your session with these three cooldown stretches (see pages 84–5 for full instructions).

Sky-reaching pose: hold for 10 seconds to 1 minute

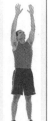

Hurdler's stretch: hold for 10 seconds to 1 minute

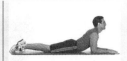

Cobra stretch: hold for 10 seconds to 1 minute

B biceps hammer

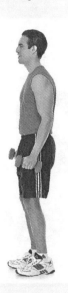

1 Stand with your feet shoulder-width apart, your back straight and your abs tight. Hold a dumbbell in each hand at your sides with your palms facing in.

2 Keeping your palms in this position, exhale as you slowly curl your arms up just past 90 degrees. Hold for 1 second. Inhale as you lower your arms to the starting position.

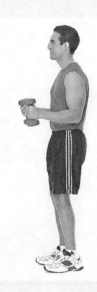

today's journal
_____ _____
_____ _____
_____ _____
_____ _____
_____ _____
_____ _____
_____ _____
_____ _____
_____ _____

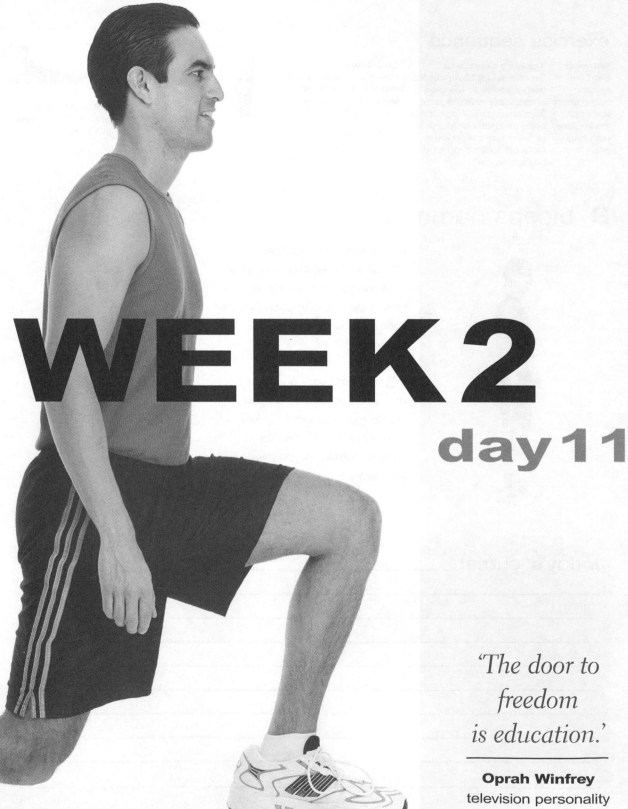

WEEK2

day 11

'The door to
freedom
is education.'

Oprah Winfrey
television personality
and actress

your wake-up talk

I show clips of the film *Cocoon* at many of my seminars to illustrate a point. The film is about a group of senior citizens whose lives are turned upside down by space aliens. At the beginning of the film, the seniors move like old people and feel unmotivated to live.

jump-start your motivation

But by the end, they move their bodies very differently – they climb trees, smile, kiss, ride bikes, jump and even dance. When they begin to move differently, they feel motivated to do anything. Moving your body differently can radically change how good you feel. Countless studies have proved that how you move your body influences your mood through your biochemistry. Hormone and oxygen levels all change with the kind of movements you make with your body. Try the exercise in 'Jump-Start Your Day'. It will have a dramatic impact on your motivation and focus.

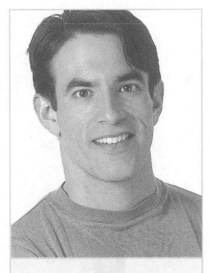

'Moving your body differently can change how you feel.'

jump-start your day

Do this exercise for at least 1 minute as often as possible throughout the day to enliven your senses. It's even better when you add some high-energy music.

1 Bring your hands together for a strong clap. With every breath, clap strongly. The palms of your hands have more nerve receptors than almost any other part of your body. Clapping your hands creates a neurological jolt that literally stimulates your brain.

2 Move into an energy posture. Stand up straight with your shoulders back and down and your chest out. This fully activates your diaphragm muscle (located under your lungs), which helps maximize your oxygen intake.

3 Jog in place. Breathe deeply as you jog in place. This further increases the rate of oxygen to your body by causing your heart to pump more blood.

today's moves
hamstrings and
quadriceps

EXERCISE LOG					
exercise	lb/kg	set 1 ✓	set 2 ✓	set 3 ✓	set 4 ✓
A					
B					

A quadriceps lunge

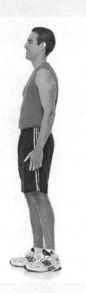

1 Stand with your feet shoulder-width apart and your arms at your sides.

2 Inhale as you step forward with your right leg until your thigh and calf form a 90-degree angle. Your right knee should not extend forward past your toes. Your left leg should also be bent to almost a 90-degree angle. Exhale as you push through your front leg to return to the starting position, then step forward with the opposite leg. Repeat 12 times with each leg.

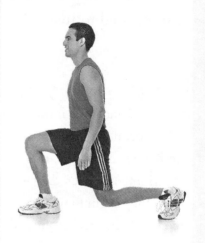

eat fat to get fit

Some people ask me if they should switch from regular processed peanut butter to the natural variety, with the oil floating on top. It's a good move because the natural variety contains fewer bad trans fats than the more processed types.

If you're going to make a change, I recommend trying almond butter instead, which can be found at health food stores and supermarkets. Most nuts are good for you, but study after study shows that almonds are among the best at fighting

heart disease and cancer. They are among the highest in omega oils. On the other hand, some research shows peanuts can be carcinogenic; fungus can be found growing in the shells, and they have fewer essential omega oils.

exercise sequence

Warmup
Start your session with a short warmup: jog in place (see page 84).

Training exercises
Do one set of 12 repetitions from exercise A, followed immediately with the same from exercise B. Repeat this cycle for a total of four sets of each exercise, checking them off on your log as you go (see box left).

Cooldown
Finish your session with these three cooldown stretches (see pages 84–5 for full instructions).

Sky-reaching pose: hold for 10 seconds to 1 minute

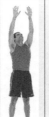

Hurdler's stretch: hold for 10 seconds to 1 minute

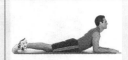

Cobra stretch: hold for 10 seconds to 1 minute

B hamstrings leg curl

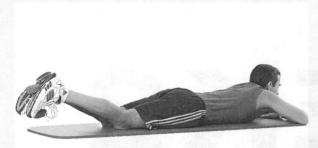

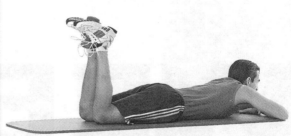

1 Lie on a mat on your stomach with your arms crossed and your chin resting on your arms. Exhale as you slowly curl your legs until your calves are at a 90-degree angle to your thighs. Hold for 1 second.

2 Inhale as you slowly lower your feet to the starting position. If you need additional resistance, wear ankle weights.

today's journal_____ _____

_____
_____
_____
_____
_____
_____
_____
_____

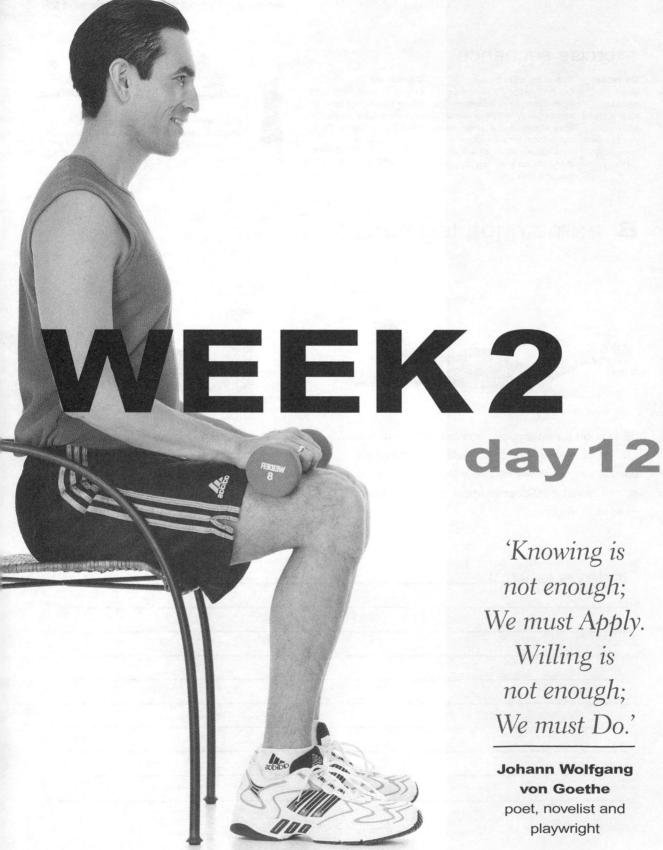

WEEK 2
day 12

'Knowing is
not enough;
We must Apply.
Willing is
not enough;
We must Do.'

**Johann Wolfgang
von Goethe**
poet, novelist and
playwright

your wake-up talk

Do you have a bad habit that you wish you could eliminate? For me it was staying up too late. I knew that the best time for me to work out was in the morning, but at the same time, I kept going to bed at 1 or 2 a.m. Of course, I would not get up until 9 or 10 a.m. This was not my goal; I wanted to be up at 5 a.m., which meant that I needed to be in bed by 10 p.m.

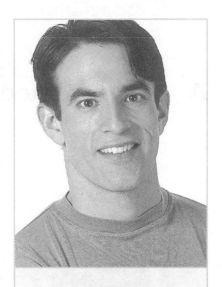

the power of replacement

To finally conquer this challenge, I had to replace the 'fulfilment' I was getting from staying up late. I used to see staying up late as bonus time to work on whatever I had not finished that day. So I replaced this bonus block of time with another block of time. Going to bed late was a waste of my time. I now see my 5 a.m. wake-up time as more efficient (I can get in a full 'East Coast' day and then a full 'West Coast' day). It gets me more excited and thus motivates me to be asleep by 10. Write down a bad habit that you want to stop. Then think about and write down what that habit has been costing you. What have you lost with this habit still in your life? Finally, come up with a replacement. It must be one that excites you as much as the old one. Write down how your life will get better with this new habit.

> 'Write down a bad habit that you want to stop.'

replacing an old habit

Old habit: _____

_____

What having this habit costs me: _____

_____

Better habit: _____

_____

What I will gain: _____

_____

today's moves
calves and
buttocks

A calves seated raise

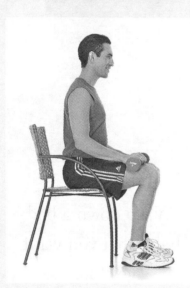

1 Sit in a sturdy chair with your feet flat on the floor and hold a dumbbell in place on top of each knee.

2 Exhale as you slowly lift your heels, keeping your toes on the floor. You should feel this in your calves. Hold for 1 second. Inhale as you lower your heels to the starting position.

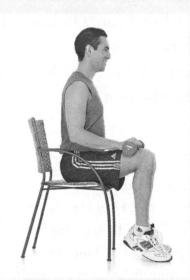

eat fat to get fit

Many of my clients (and many of you!) love butter. And most people don't want to give it up. There is room for all foods in the Eat Fat to Get Fit food plan, including butter, but I want you to try a simple switch for a few days. Fill a small plastic container with olive oil and put it in the refrigerator. The oil will harden, taking on the consistency of butter. Spread this on your toast instead of butter. It *will* taste different at first, but after a few days, your taste buds will grow used to it, and you'll actually come to prefer the olive oil.

exercise sequence

Warmup
Start your session with a short warmup: jog in place (see page 84).

Training exercises
Do one set of 12 repetitions from exercise A, followed immediately with the same from exercise B. Repeat this cycle for a total of four sets of each exercise, checking them off on your log as you go (see box left).

Cooldown
Finish your session with these three cooldown stretches (see pages 84–5 for full instructions).

Sky-reaching pose: hold for 10 seconds to 1 minute

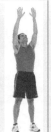

Hurdler's stretch: hold for 10 seconds to 1 minute

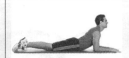

Cobra stretch: hold for 10 seconds to 1 minute

B buttocks squeeze

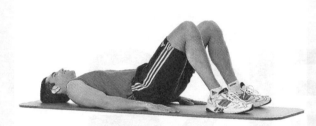

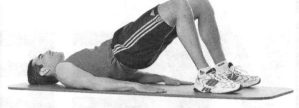

1 Lie on a mat on your back with your palms flat on the mat, your feet shoulder-width apart and your knees bent.

2 Exhale as you press through your feet to lift your buttocks 3 to 6 in (7 to 15 cm) off the floor. Push your pelvis up, flattening the natural S-curve in your lower back. Squeeze your buttocks for 1 second. Inhale as you slowly return to the starting position.

today's journal _____ _____

_____ _____

_____ _____

_____ _____

_____ _____

_____ _____

_____ _____

_____ _____

_____ _____

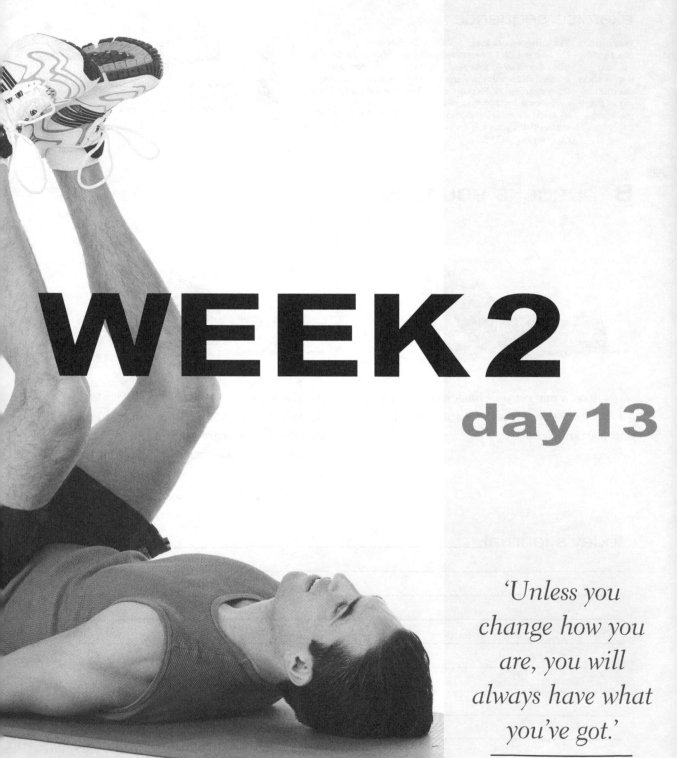

WEEK2
day 13

'Unless you change how you are, you will always have what you've got.'

Jim Rohn
business philosopher

your wake-up talk

Today's Wake-Up Talk is simple and fun. Rewards are powerful motivators, so I want you to think of something you can give yourself at the end of your 28-Day Challenge.

create a reward for yourself

Remember, your reward must be something you love and at the same time must be something that supports your new lifestyle. It must also be consistent with the new person you are becoming.

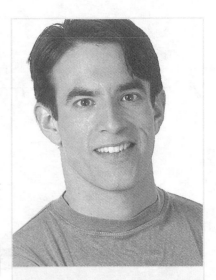

my reward

Here is a list of some simple rewards.

- New outfit
- A day at the beach
- A day at a spa
- Romantic dinner for two
- Tickets to a show or concert
- A new piece of sports equipment, such as a new bike or golf clubs

Pick something you really would love to give yourself and write it down. After you choose your reward, tell a friend or your partner. If you can afford it, invite them as well. By getting them in on your reward, you get them to help you stay accountable and on track.

'Think of something you can give yourself as a reward.'

today's moves
inner thigh and
outer thigh

EXERCISE LOG					
exercise	lb/kg	set 1 ✓	set 2 ✓	set 3 ✓	set 4 ✓
A					
B					

A inner thigh frog

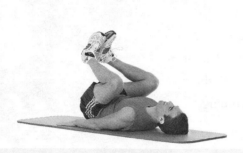 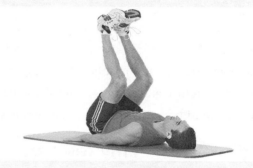

1 Lie on a mat on your back with your palms flat on the mat by your sides. Pull your knees into your chest. Allow your feet to touch and your knees to splay to the sides, resembling a frog's leg position.

2 Exhale as you raise your legs straight up, keeping the inner edges of your feet together. Stop before your legs are completely straight, making sure not to lock your knees. Hold for 1 second. Inhale as you return to the starting position.

eat fat to get fit

The protein in dairy products, called casein, is an allergen that can cause asthma and sinus problems. I can vouch for that; as soon as I cut most of the dairy out of my diet, my headaches and asthma went away.

If you love to pour milk on your cereal and eat sandwiches with cheese, try switching to soya products. For every dairy product you can think of, there is a soya substitute. There are soya versions of milk, cheese, sour

cream, butter, yoghurt and even ice cream. No, they don't all taste exactly like the real thing, but often, they taste better. And they are better for you. Sample different brands until you find ones that you enjoy.

exercise sequence

Warmup
Start your session with a short warmup: jog in place (see page 84).

Training exercises
Do one set of 12 repetitions from exercise A, followed immediately with the same from exercise B. Repeat this cycle for a total of four sets of each exercise, checking them off on your log as you go (see box left).

Cooldown
Finish your session with these three cooldown stretches (see pages 84–5 for full instructions).

Sky-reaching pose: hold for 10 seconds to 1 minute

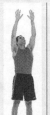

Hurdler's stretch: hold for 10 seconds to 1 minute

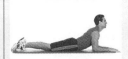

Cobra stretch: hold for 10 seconds to 1 minute

B outer thigh leg raise

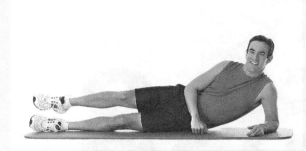

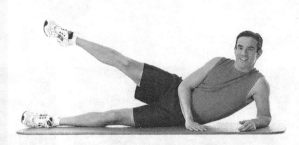

1 Lie on a mat on your left side. Support your upper body with your left elbow. Your legs should be extended and aligned with your upper body.

2 Exhale as you slowly raise your upper leg. Hold for 1 second. Inhale as you slowly lower your leg to the starting position. Repeat 12 times with your left leg, then switch sides. For more resistance, wear ankle weights.

today's journal _____ _____

_____ _____

_____ _____

_____ _____

_____ _____

_____ _____

_____ _____

_____ _____

_____ _____

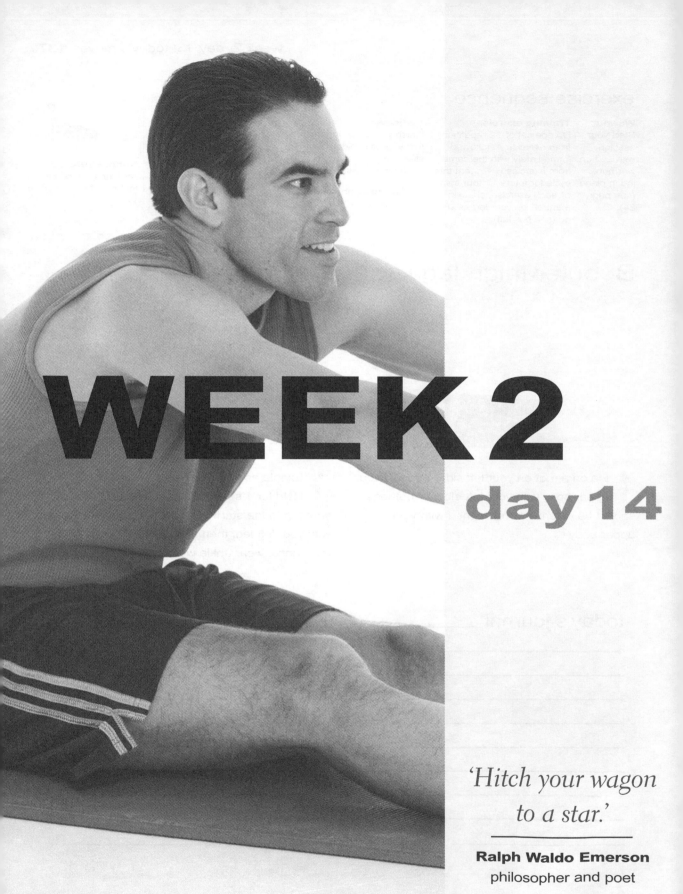

WEEK 2
day 14

'Hitch your wagon
to a star.'

Ralph Waldo Emerson
philosopher and poet

your wake-up talk

How do you feel when you are in the dark? Most people slow down and become tired. It's a biological fact: for thousands of years, the human race has gone to sleep when it's dark and has woken up when it's light.

use the power of light

You can use light to your advantage to stay focused and motivated throughout your day. Start using the power of light as soon as you wake up so that you feel your best during your 8 Minutes in the Morning workout. Adding more light to your day radically improves your mood and mental state, according to Dr Bob Arnot, author of *The Biology of Success*.

Go through the checklist in 'Bright Ideas' and start to incorporate as many as you can into your environment at home and at work. I guarantee that you will feel sharper and more motivated throughout the day. Then you'll continue to take the actions that will get you lean.

This is your day off, so take some extra time for yourself. Go for a powerwalk, get some fresh air and motivate yourself for next week.

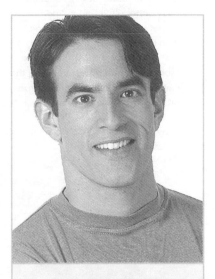

'Use light to stay focused throughout your day.'

bright ideas

- Change all of your home lighting to 100-watt bulbs.
- Go outside for a few minutes each day.
- Arrange your home to take advantage of open windows
- Leave your blinds up or curtains open at night so that the sunlight will wake you naturally in the morning.

Note: If you would like to learn about light therapy, visit *www.sunboxco.com* and *www.sltbr.org*.

8 minute marvel Tony lost 1st 6 lb (9 kg)!

I was having a hard time finding balance in my diet and exercise routine because of my seriously busy schedule. I had to find something that was simple and didn't take a lot of time. I found that with Jorge's 8 Minutes in the Morning programme, just doing the exercises and eating right put me on the road to better health.

Tony Natoli
Salesman

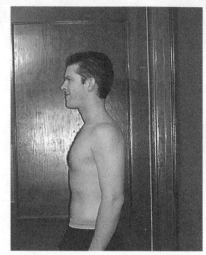

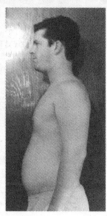

before

'It also gave me the right mindset to achieve all of the little successes that people in sales encounter on a daily basis.'

eat fat to get fit

If you like chocolate, you'll be happy to know that your body treats cocoa butter the same way it does olive oil.

The good news is chocolate does not raise blood cholesterol and can even improve your blood cholesterol profile.

But there's a catch: milk chocolate contains butterfat. Unlike other forms of chocolate, milk chocolate with butterfat can raise your blood cholesterol levels. It also contains very little cocoa compared to the more bitter dark chocolate. Cheaper chocolates often replace the cocoa butter with bad fats like palm oil or even partially hydrogenated oils.

So if you're going to eat chocolate, buy dark chocolate made from cocoa butter and no fillers.

IMPORTANT: WEEK 2 UPDATE

It's time to monitor how you are doing and record your second week's progress. This will keep you focused and accountable. Grab a pen and answer the following questions.

1 What is your current weight? Use scales to weigh yourself and also write down your original weight.

    _____

2 What have you done well this week? What makes you proud of you? _____

    _____

    _____

    _____

    _____

3 What could you be doing better or improving?

    _____

    _____

    _____

    _____

    _____

4 What is your game plan for week 3? _____

    _____

    _____

    _____

    _____

Interact with
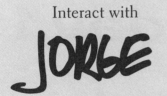

If you would like me to contact you about your progress, send me an e-mail with your answers to this week's update to *weektwo@jorgecruise.com*. I will send you a special e-mail with bonus tips on how to make week 3 even more fun and effective.

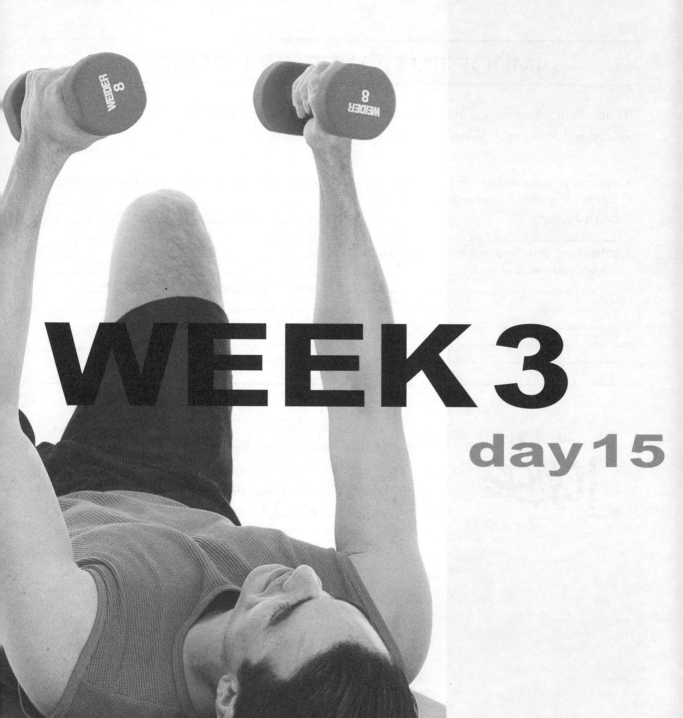

WEEK 3

day 15

'*Follow your bliss.*'

Joseph Campbell
author of *The Power
of Myth*

your wake-up talk

Think of a film you really love. Chances are it'll have a soundtrack that dramatically enhances it. Without music, most films would not have the powerful emotion and energy that we all love. The same is true for getting a lean body. Music improves your workouts simply because humans are rhythmic souls; we naturally crave a beat to follow. Your heart has rhythm to it; your breathing pattern has rhythm to it. Once a beat starts, you want to start moving.

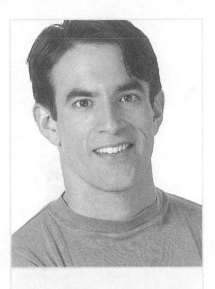

the power of music

Music is magic and will make your 8 Minutes in the Morning workout much more enjoyable, guaranteed. The secret to using music is that it must have a continuous percussive beat so you naturally want to move.

Latin music is my pick; that percussive beat is the heart and pulse of almost all Latin music. So, go out and buy yourself some new music. It can be Latin, but more important, it must be music you love.

'Go out and buy yourself some new music.'

great songs to get you moving

Working out to music is the perfect way to start the day. To help you get moving, I have selected some of my favourite songs that I love to exercise to. These music hits from the '70s, '80s, '90s and today are recorded at 126 beats per minute (BPM), the perfect pace to complement your daily 8 Minutes in the Morning routine! Listen to them on my website, go to *www.jorgecruise.com/music*.

today's moves
chest and
back

EXERCISE LOG					
exercise	lb/kg	set 1 ✓	set 2 ✓	set 3 ✓	set 4 ✓
A					
B					

A chest fly

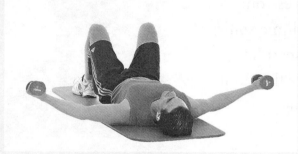 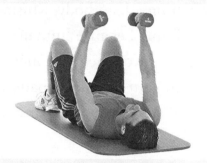

1 Lie on a mat on your back with your knees bent and your feet flat on the floor. With a dumbbell in each hand, extend your arms straight out from your body on the floor, palms facing up.

2 Exhale as you slowly raise your arms straight up so that the dumbbells are almost touching each other above your chest. Your palms should be facing each other. Keep your elbows slightly bent. Hold for 1 second. Inhale as you slowly lower your arms to the starting position.

eat fat to get fit

Is the rest of your family turning up their noses at your efforts to add more vegetables to meals? Then sneak them in. That's right: with a little creativity, you'll all be eating more vegetables without them noticing.

The secret to sneaking vegetables into family meals is to cut them into very small pieces and mix them into dishes that don't normally contain them. For example, you can mix chopped onions, peppers, carrots and cabbage into meat loaf, or purée some vegetables and add them to pasta sauce. You can also add small vegetable chunks to your next casserole. The possibilities are endless.

exercise sequence

Warmup
Start your session with a short warmup: jog in place (see page 84).

Training exercises
Do one set of 12 repetitions from exercise A, followed immediately with the same from exercise B. Repeat this cycle for a total of four sets of each exercise, checking them off on your log as you go (see box left).

Cooldown
Finish your session with these three cooldown stretches (see pages 84–5 for full instructions).

Sky-reaching pose: hold for 10 seconds to 1 minute

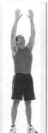

Hurdler's stretch: hold for 10 seconds to 1 minute

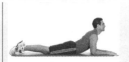

Cobra stretch: hold for 10 seconds to 1 minute

B back standing bent-over row

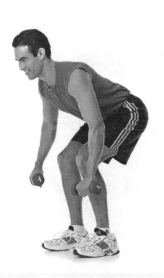

1 Stand with your feet shoulder-width apart. With a dumbbell in each hand, bend over so that your backside sticks out and your knees are bent. Extend your arms so that your hands are directly beneath your shoulders.

2 Keeping your back straight, exhale as you slowly bring your elbows straight back, pulling the dumbbells towards your chest. Hold for 1 second. Inhale as you lower the dumbbells to the starting position.

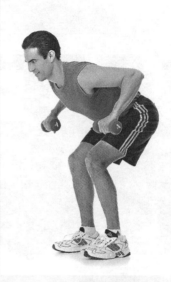

today's journal _____

_____ _____

_____ _____

_____ _____

_____ _____

_____ _____

_____ _____

_____ _____

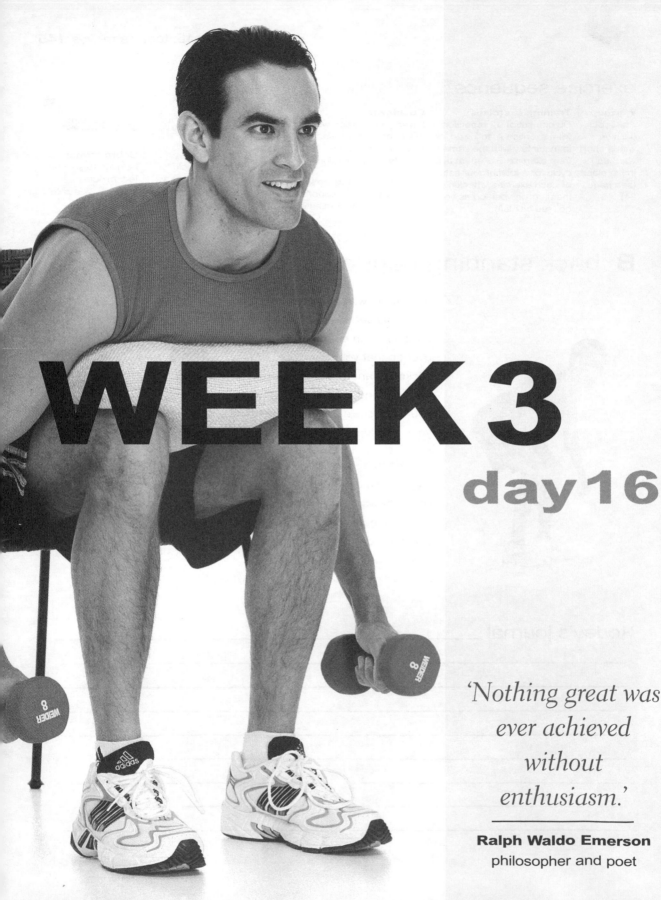

WEEK 3
day 16

'Nothing great was
ever achieved
without
enthusiasm.'

Ralph Waldo Emerson
philosopher and poet

your wake-up talk

What if you could use your everyday breathing as a powerful tool to boost your energy and motivation? Breath is the key to increasing your energy and focus because it is the only way that you can bring oxygen into your body. Without enough oxygen, you become lethargic, tired and depressed. With increased oxygen levels, you not only increase your energy but also dramatically improve your mood. You simply feel better.

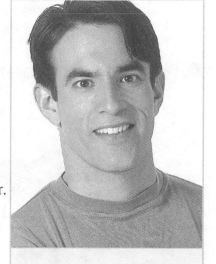

breathe deep and feel great

The secret to making your breathing more effective is learning how to 'belly breathe'. People in India have been doing this for hundreds of years. Belly breathing is the primary foundation for yoga and it is easy to learn. You will love how it makes you feel.

The key to belly breathing is using your diaphragm, a dome-shaped muscle located under your lungs. When you draw it outward (pushing your belly forward), it opens your lungs, drawing oxygen in. And when you push it inward by contracting your belly, you effectively move the used oxygen out of your lungs.

Try to use this type of breathing all day today, especially when you feel tired and lethargic.

'Learn how to belly breathe.'

belly breathing for energy

1 Stand up straight with your shoulders pulled back and your chest pushed out.

2 Inhale through your nose for a count of 4 (make sure that your belly comes out), and hold for a count of 2.

3 Exhale through your mouth for a count of 5 (make sure that your belly contracts by coming inward).

4 Repeat for a total of 10 deep breaths. Do this whenever you feel worn out, especially when you think that you're too tired to exercise.

today's moves
shoulders and
abdominals

A shoulders bent-over lateral raise

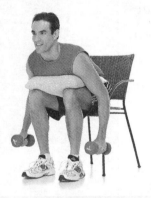 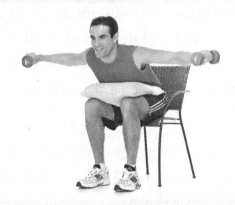

1 Sit in a sturdy chair and grasp a dumbbell in each hand. You may put a pillow on your lap for support. Lean forward, making sure to keep your back straight. Your arms should be slightly bent at your sides.

2 Exhale as you slowly raise the dumbbells to your sides, keeping your elbows slightly bent. Hold for 1 second. Inhale as you slowly return to the starting position.

eat fat to get fit

As I mentioned earlier, saturated fat is one of the worst fats you can eat.

One way to lower your intake of saturated fat is to switch from red meat such as beef to white meat such as chicken or turkey, which contains 33 to 80 per cent less fat than beef. And of the fat in poultry, less of it is the saturated type than in beef.

But don't stop there. Most of the fat in chicken and turkey is found in and just underneath the skin. If you eat chicken with the skin, you double the amount of fat.

Fortunately, even without its skin, chicken and turkey are still high in quality protein, B vitamins, iron and zinc.

exercise sequence

Warmup
Start your session with a short warmup: jog in place (see page 84).

Training exercises
Do one set of 12 repetitions from exercise A, followed immediately with the same from exercise B. Repeat this cycle for a total of four sets of each exercise, checking them off on your log as you go (see box left).

Cooldown
Finish your session with these three cooldown stretches (see pages 84–5 for full instructions).

Sky-reaching pose: hold for 10 seconds to 1 minute

Hurdler's stretch: hold for 10 seconds to 1 minute

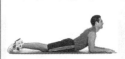

Cobra stretch: hold for 10 seconds to 1 minute

B abdominals crunch

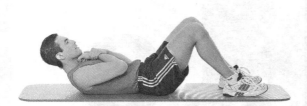

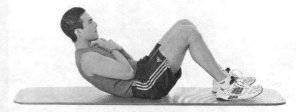

1 Lie on a mat on your back with your knees bent and your feet flat on the floor. Make a fist with one hand and place it between your chin and collarbone. With your other hand, grasp your wrist. This will prevent you from leading with your head and straining your neck.

2 Without moving your lower body, exhale and slowly curl your upper torso until your shoulder blades are off the ground. Hold for 1 second. Inhale as you slowly lower yourself to the starting position.

today's journal_____ _____

_____ _____
_____ _____
_____ _____
_____ _____
_____ _____
_____ _____
_____ _____
_____ _____

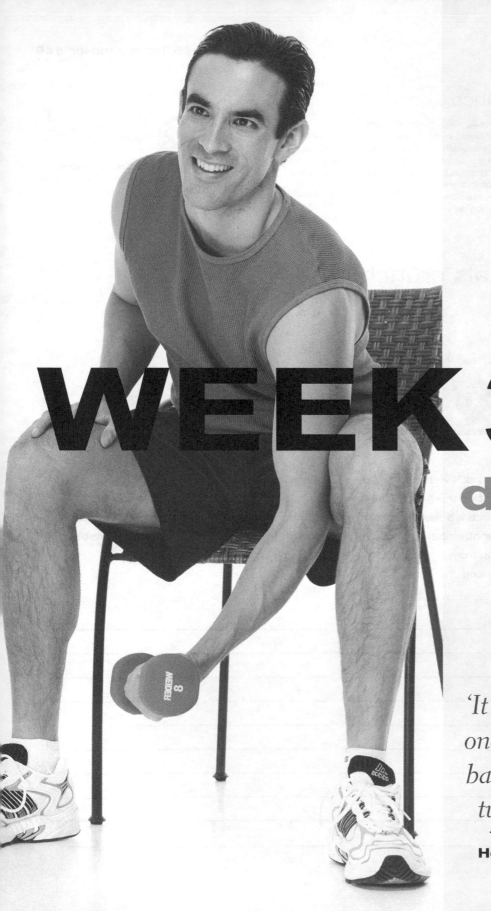

WEEK3
day 17

'It is as hard to see
one's self as to look
backwards without
turning around.'

Henry David Thoreau
writer

your wake-up talk

Having been through a challenging health crisis – and watching members of my family go through challenging health crises – I can tell you that becoming physically reborn is completely fulfilling. And nothing in life is as amazing as finishing something you set your heart on. It takes focus and dedication, yet nothing is as satisfying as changing your body and your life. But starting an important project such as getting fit and not seeing it through is burdening. It drains you.

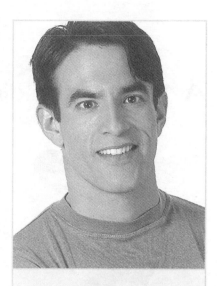

'Nothing in life is as amazing as finishing something you set your heart on.'

be a finisher

My advice to you is to continue to take the higher road and be a finisher. The rewards are worth it. To increase your success, write down three difficult projects that you have finished. Examples include leaving school or college, landing your first job or buying your first home. Get excited because *you are a finisher*. You *will* achieve your dream body.

Then write down the three worst things that will happen to you if you don't finish the programme and get lean. Look 5 years from now, then 10 years from now. How bad will your life become? Use this dissatisfaction to push you to the finish.

focus on finishing

3 Projects I Have Finished Successfully
1 _____
2 _____
3 _____

3 Worst Things That Will Happen if I Don't Get Lean
1 _____
2 _____
3 _____

today's moves
triceps and
biceps

EXERCISE LOG					
exercise	lb/kg	set 1 ✓	set 2 ✓	set 3 ✓	set 4 ✓
A					
B					

A triceps standing kickback

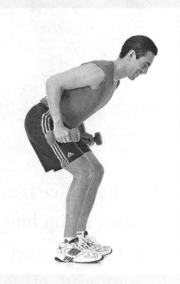 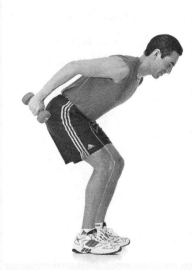

1 Stand with your feet shoulder-width apart, your knees bent and a dumbbell in each hand. Bend forward slightly, keeping your back straight and abs tight. Bend your arms at a 90-degree angle.

2 Exhale as you slowly straighten your arms and press the dumbbells behind your buttocks, keeping your elbows slightly bent. Hold for 1 second. Inhale as you slowly return to the starting position.

eat fat to get fit

For many people, numerous unneeded calories come from what I call mindless eating. This happens any time you eat while doing something else such as driving, watching television or surfing the Internet. Because your attention is elsewhere, you don't really taste your food or even register that you've eaten it. So you tend to eat much more than you normally would have.

If you want to chew on something while doing another task, I suggest sugar-free chewing gum. Research shows that chewing gum can actually burn a handful of extra calories a day. But the best part is that it keeps your mouth busy. You can also try drinking lots of water or munching on low-calorie snacks such as celery sticks and cucumber slices.

exercise sequence

Warmup
Start your session with a short warmup: jog in place (see page 84).

Training exercises
Do one set of 12 repetitions from exercise A, followed immediately with the same from exercise B. Repeat this cycle for a total of four sets of each exercise, checking them off on your log as you go (see box left).

Cooldown
Finish your session with these three cooldown stretches (see pages 84–5 for full instructions).

Sky-reaching pose: hold for 10 seconds to 1 minute

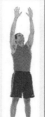

Hurdler's stretch: hold for 10 seconds to 1 minute

Cobra stretch: hold for 10 seconds to 1 minute

B biceps one-arm curl

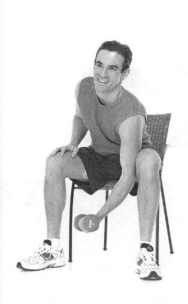

1 Sit in a sturdy chair and hold a dumbbell in your left hand. Bend forward and extend your left arm between your legs so that your elbow is braced against the inside of your left thigh.

2 Exhale as you curl the dumbbell, bringing your palm towards your bicep. When you've curled your arm just beyond a 90-degree angle, hold for 1 second. Inhale as you lower the dumbbell to the starting position. Repeat 12 times with the same arm, then switch sides.

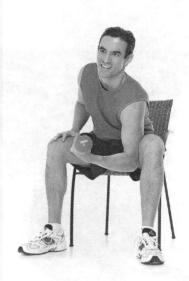

today's journal

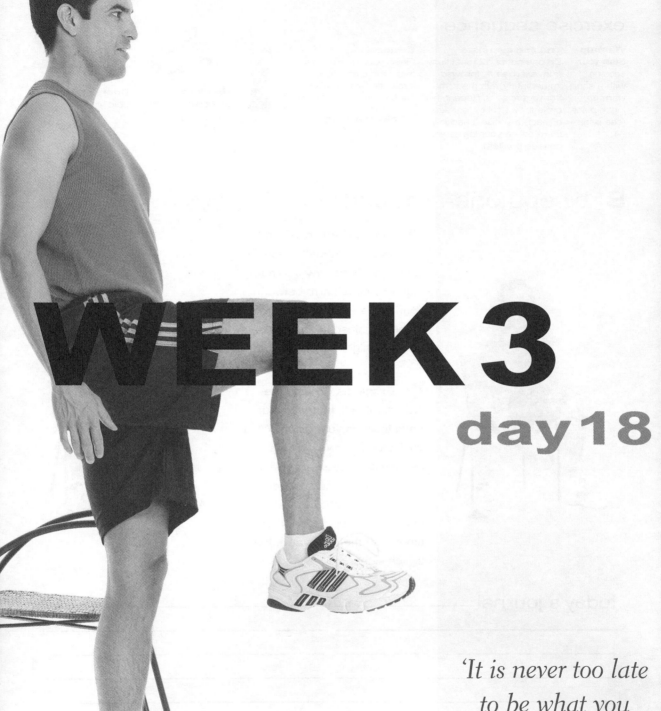

WEEK 3
day 18

'It is never too late
to be what you
might have been.'

George Eliot
novelist

your wake-up talk

In the process of coaching more than 3 million people online, I've discovered the most effective tricks to staying on track for the long term. It's all about knowing how to direct your focus. Your focus determines what you see and hear, which affects how you feel. How you feel determines your behaviour.

focus on the positive

This morning's Wake-Up Talk teaches you the most powerful technique you can use to immediately change your focus from negative to positive. By using this technique, you will instantly start to change how you feel. It's what I call the Master Question. (Recall the power of Result-Driven Questions from Week 1 Day 5.) You need to ask yourself the Master Question over and over again, almost like a mantra. Say it out loud or to yourself to focus your mind on success. This Master Question is simple and will immediately direct your focus on what you will gain. The more you use it, the stronger your motivation will become. Remember: if you ask, you shall receive.

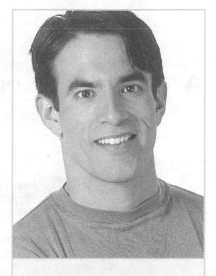

'If you ask, you shall receive.'

the master question

The more you ask yourself this question, the stronger your motivation will become. Use it every morning and throughout the day. I guarantee it will give you a powerful advantage in staying motivated long term!

The Master Question: How great will my life become once I am fit?

today's moves
hamstrings and
quadriceps

EXERCISE LOG					
exercise	lb/kg	set 1 ✓	set 2 ✓	set 3 ✓	set 4 ✓
A					
B					

A hamstrings one-leg curl

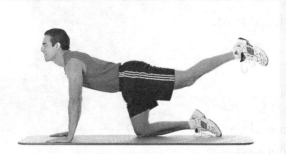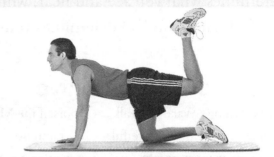

1 Kneel on a mat on all fours with your knees hip-width apart, your hands placed slightly wider than your shoulders and your fingers pointing forward. With your head up, raise your left leg, keeping your leg extended.

2 Once your foot is level with your buttocks, exhale as you slowly curl your foot to form a 90-degree angle with your buttocks. Hold for 1 second. Inhale as you lower your foot to the starting position. Repeat 12 times with the left leg, then switch sides.

eat fat to get fit

Tuna, chicken, prawns and crab are all great-tasting low-saturated-fat choices of quality protein. But sometimes the way these foods are prepared can nearly destroy their healthy reputation. For instance, tuna, chicken and seafood salads are all made with lots of mayonnaise, one of the worse condiments because it is high in cholesterol and saturated fat. If you love tuna and chicken salad sandwiches, you do have an option. Make them by mixing the meat or seafood with soya mayonnaise, which can be found in health food shops and some supermarkets. It contains none of the saturated fat of regular mayonnaise, but has all of the health benefits of soya.

exercise sequence

Warmup
Start your session with a short warmup: jog in place (see page 84).

Training exercises
Do one set of 12 repetitions from exercise A, followed immediately with the same from exercise B. Repeat this cycle for a total of four sets of each exercise, checking them off on your log as you go (see box left).

Cooldown
Finish your session with these three cooldown stretches (see pages 84–5 for full instructions).

Sky-reaching pose: hold for 10 seconds to 1 minute

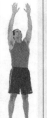

Hurdler's stretch: hold for 10 seconds to 1 minute

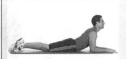

Cobra stretch: hold for 10 seconds to 1 minute

B quadriceps standing raise

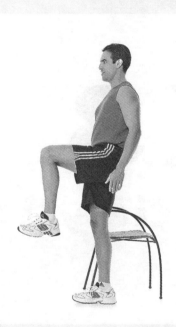

1 Stand with your feet shoulder-width apart and your arms at your sides. Shift your body weight to your right leg and raise your left foot until your left leg is bent at the knee at a 90-degree angle. (If you feel unbalanced, hold on to a sturdy chair.)

2 Exhale as you slowly extend your left foot forward. Hold for 1 second. Inhale as you lower your foot to the starting position. Repeat 12 times with the left leg, then switch sides.

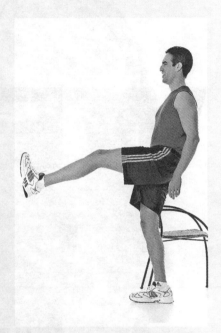

today's journal

_____ _____
_____ _____
_____ _____
_____ _____
_____ _____
_____ _____
_____ _____
_____ _____
_____ _____

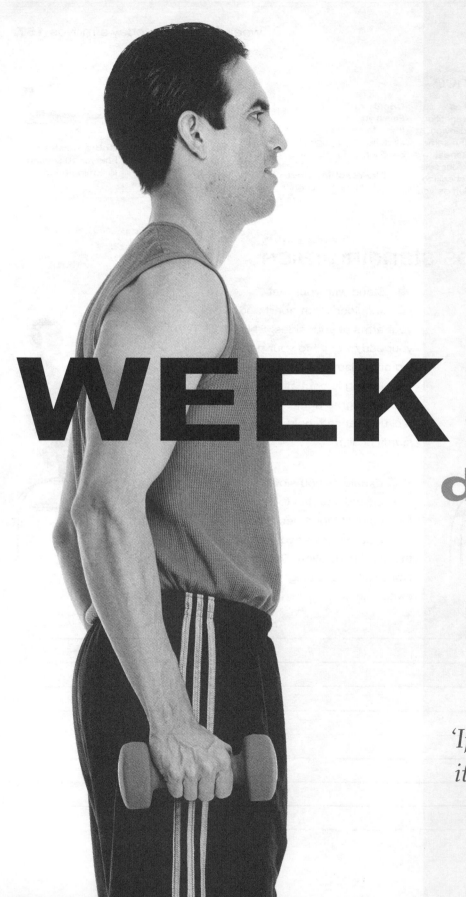

WEEK 3
day 19

'If you can dream
it, you can do it.'

Walt Disney
filmmaker and
animator

your wake-up talk

Today I want to share with you a simple trick that will help you change your mood for the better, jump-starting your motivation. The key is to change your brain's chemistry by naturally increasing the levels of a special neurotransmitter called serotonin. Research at the University of California at Los Angeles has demonstrated that higher amounts of serotonin in our brains make us feel better, while lower amounts make us feel depressed and scattered.

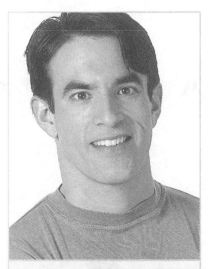

feel extraordinary with serotonin

The key to maximizing serotonin is not found at the chemist or in Prozac or St John's wort. It's in a smile.

Research shows that you can literally increase the amount of serotonin in your brain by changing your facial expression. For example, by smiling, you change the flow of blood to your brain and provide an internal environment ideal for producing serotonin. So if you want to feel better immediately, just smile.

'If you want to feel better, just smile.'

give yourself a reason to smile

List 5 to 10 things that make you smile, from a heartwarming memory to a funny joke to sunshine on your face. Read your list whenever you need some help with your smile. How has a simple smile changed your life?

1 _____
2 _____
3 _____
4 _____
5 _____

6 _____
7 _____
8 _____
9 _____
10 _____

today's moves
calves and
buttocks

EXERCISE LOG					
exercise	lb/kg	set 1 ✓	set 2 ✓	set 3 ✓	set 4 ✓
A					
B					

A calves heel raise

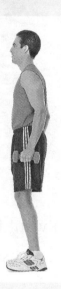

1 Stand with your feet shoulder-width apart. Hold a dumbbell in each hand at your sides, with your arms extended but not locked. Keep your chest out, your shoulder blades rolled back and down and your abs tight.

2 Exhale as you slowly lift your heels, rising onto your tiptoes. Hold for 1 second. Inhale as you slowly lower yourself back to the starting position.

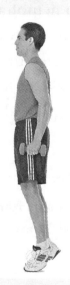

eat fat to get fit

I remember when the bagel craze was at its peak, with bagel-and-coffee shops everywhere I went. People couldn't seem to get enough of these treats. But what really amazes me is the reputation that bagels erroneously earned for being a healthy food.

While bagels are low in fat, they are not necessarily low in calories. A typical bagel contains a whopping 400 calories and accounts for 4 Complex Carbohydrate boxes on your Eating Cards. Worse, many toppings, such as cream cheese and butter, are high in

unhealthy saturated fat.

That doesn't mean that you have to give up bagels completely, but I do recommend that you restrict yourself to eating half of a medium-size bagel, which amounts to just 1 Complex Carbohydrate box on your Eating Cards.

exercise sequence

Warmup
Start your session with a short warmup: jog in place (see page 84).

Training exercises
Do one set of 12 repetitions from exercise A, followed immediately with the same from exercise B. Repeat this cycle for a total of four sets of each exercise, checking them off on your log as you go (see box left).

Cooldown
Finish your session with these three cooldown stretches (see pages 84–5 for full instructions).

Sky-reaching pose: hold for 10 seconds to 1 minute

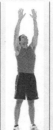

Hurdler's stretch: hold for 10 seconds to 1 minute

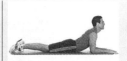
Cobra stretch: hold for 10 seconds to 1 minute

B buttocks leg lift

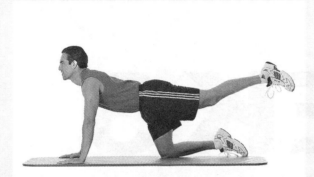

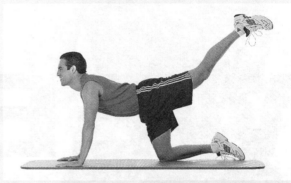

1 Kneel on a mat on all fours with your knees hip-width apart, your hands placed slightly wider than your shoulders and your fingers pointing forward. With your head up, raise your left leg and extend your knee until your leg is parallel to the floor.

2 Exhale as you slowly bring your whole leg up as high as you can. Focus on moving only from your hip. If this puts too much stress on your back, lower your head so that you are looking down at the mat. Hold for 1 second. Inhale as you slowly return to the starting position. Repeat 12 times with the left leg, then switch sides.

today's journal

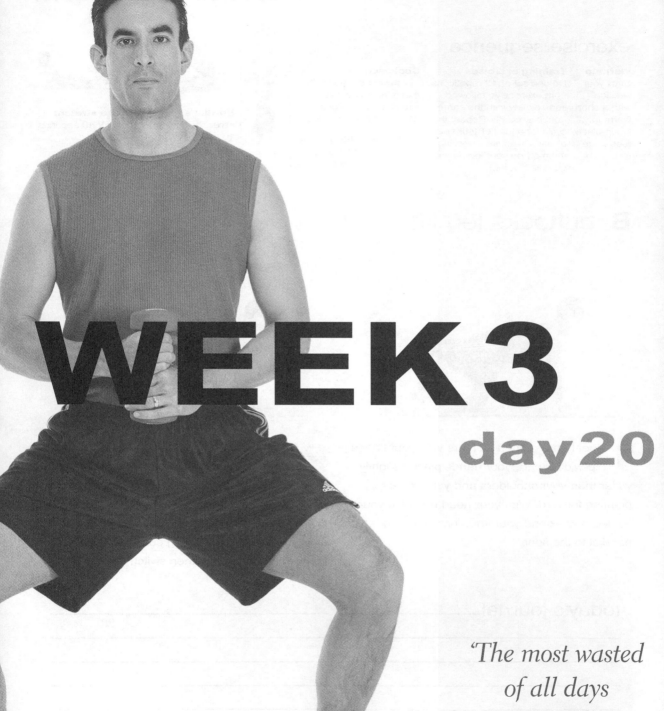

WEEK 3
day 20

'The most wasted
of all days
is one without
laughter.'

e e cummings
poet

your wake-up talk

Words and phrases can powerfully and instantly affect how you feel about things. You may remember from English class that a metaphor is a way to indirectly describe what something means. For example: 'I am floating on air', 'I am stuck between a rock and a hard place', and 'I am at the end of my tether'. You use a metaphor whenever you explain a concept by linking it to something else.

find metaphors that get you lean

Here is the key: when you use a metaphor, you also are taking on the rules and preconceived notions that accompany that metaphor. In other words, the metaphors you use directly affect how you feel. If you use an empowering one, you will feel empowered. For example, instead of referring to exercise as a chore or work, think of it as a gift or as play.

I've already come up with six power metaphors to help keep me (and you!) motivated to get lean.

'Words can powerfully affect how you feel about things.'

my power metaphors

Use these power metaphors to stay motivated. If you think of others, e-mail the best ones to me at *metaphors@jorgecruise.com*.

My body is the most precious instrument I will ever own.

Food is fuel.

Exercise is a gift.

Life is a game.

My body is the temple for my soul.

Food is my medicine.

today's moves
inner thigh and
outer thigh

EXERCISE LOG					
exercise	lb/kg	set 1 ✓	set 2 ✓	set 3 ✓	set 4 ✓
A					
B					

A inner thigh plié

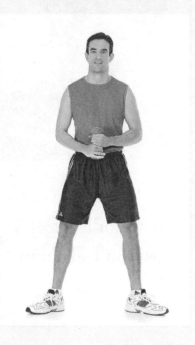 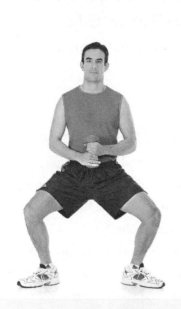

1 Stand with your feet slightly wider than shoulder-width apart. Point your toes away from the centre of your body and point your heels inwards. Grasp a dumbbell with both hands in front of your abdomen.

2 Exhale as you squat down until your knees are bent almost at a 90-degree angle. If your knees extend forward past your toes, your feet are not far enough apart. Hold for 1 second. Inhale as you slowly rise to the starting position.

eat fat to get fit

It's hard to watch your portions when you eat out. Restaurants routinely serve huge meals that can easily add up to 1,000 calories or more. And everything looks and tastes so good that it's hard to keep yourself from eating everything on your plate, even when you feel your tummy bulging against your belt.

If you're with a friend, ask her to remind you to eat slowly and taste your food. It's a simple trick, but you'll actually eat less automatically because you'll be paying attention to what you're putting in your mouth. Also, as soon as your meal arrives, you can cut your portions in half and wrap up the extra food in a take-home container before you are tempted to eat it. Check out other great tips in 'Eating Fit at Restaurants' on page 79.

exercise sequence

Warmup
Start your session with a short warmup: jog in place (see page 84).

Training exercises
Do one set of 12 repetitions from exercise A, followed immediately with the same from exercise B. Repeat this cycle for a total of four sets of each exercise, checking them off on your log as you go (see box left).

Cooldown
Finish your session with these three cooldown stretches (see pages 84–5 for full instructions).

Sky-reaching pose: hold for 10 seconds to 1 minute

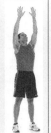

Hurdler's stretch: hold for 10 seconds to 1 minute

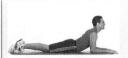

Cobra stretch: hold for 10 seconds to 1 minute

B outer thigh pep leader

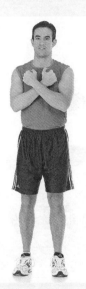

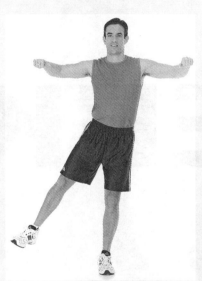

1 Stand with your feet shoulder-width apart and your arms crossed over your chest. Exhale as you lift your right leg out to the side and extend your arms for balance. Hold for 1 second.

2 Inhale as you slowly lower your leg to the starting position. Repeat 12 times with the right leg, then switch sides.

today's journal _____ _____

_____ _____

_____ _____

_____ _____

_____ _____

_____ _____

_____ _____

_____ _____

_____ _____

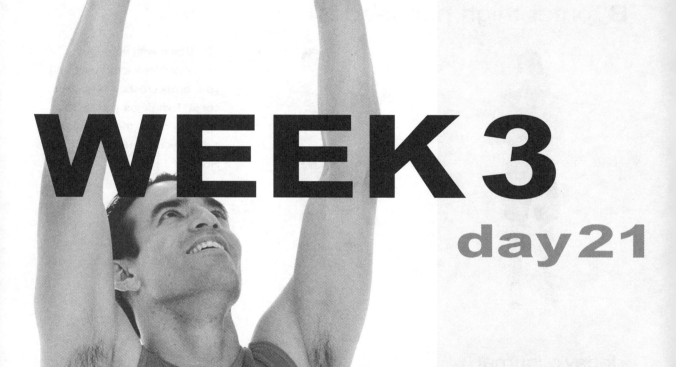

WEEK3
day21

'Shoot for the moon. Even if you miss, you'll land among the stars.'

Les Brown
motivational author

your wake-up talk

One of the most important secrets that will directly affect the quality of your health, fitness and life is the idea that who you spend time with is who you become. It is probably the most valuable lesson I have learned in my life.

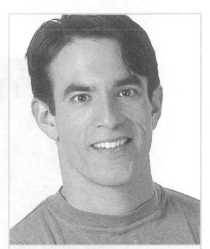

'It is critical to create some sort of support team.'

you are who you spend time with

So when people ask me if they should join a gym or fitness club, I tell them that it is not necessary, but that it is critical to create some sort of support team. That could be a gym or fitness club, an online weight-loss chat group (such as the one at *www.jorgecruise.com*), a recreation or sports centre, a healthy cooking class or even a fitness book club.

The key is to seek out people who are living life at the highest level, especially in regard to fitness and health. You want to surround yourself with people who are like-minded and interested in getting fitter.

This is critical. It will help change your life!

This is your day off, so take some extra time for yourself. Go for a powerwalk, get some fresh air and motivate yourself for next week.

my support teams

Often, we don't achieve the best we are capable of because we put ourselves in an environment that never encourages us to be our best. Write down the names of people who support you, encourage you and bring out your best, then make time to visit these people on a regular basis. Also write down new places and environments that can help you meet more supportive people.

People who already support me: _____

_____

_____

New places/environments to support me: _____

_____

_____

8 minute marvel Jill lost 15 lb (7.5 kg)!

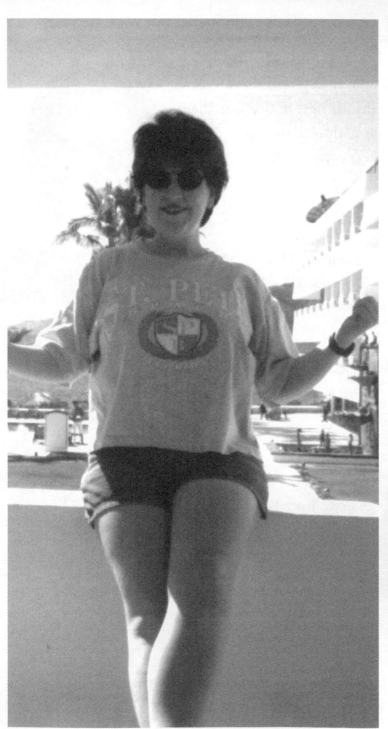

When I first started 8 Minutes in the Morning, I weighed 10 st 10 lb (68 kg) and felt unfit and fatigued. I had tried every diet out there and nothing had worked for me. But each week during 8 Minutes in the Morning, I lost an average of 2 lb (1kg).

'As time went by, I could feel my posture improving.'

I was soon standing straighter and had more bounce in my walk. I feel terrific and I look forward to my workouts every morning; they help me start my day off on the right track.

Jill Leonard
Telephone Service Representative

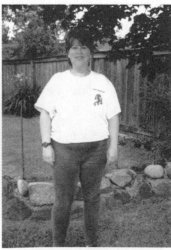

before

eat fat to get fit

To start eating better, all you need to do is turn on your computer. You'll find a treasure trove of information on the Internet, with literally hundreds of helpful food and nutrition sites that can help you meet your goals.

www.drweil.com This site is a great resource for information on vitamins, herbs, supplements and alternative medicine.

www.nutrition.org.uk Maintained by the British Nutrition Foundation, this site offers up-to-date information on the latest food trends.

www.organicsdirect.co.uk. This e-commerce site will deliver fresh organic produce to your door.

IMPORTANT: WEEK 3 UPDATE

It's time to see how you are doing and record your third week's progress. This will keep you focused and accountable. Grab a pen and answer the following questions.

1 What is your current weight? Use scales to weigh yourself and also write down your original weight.

_____

2 What have you done well this week? What makes you proud of you? _____

_____

_____

_____

_____

_____

3 What could you be doing better or improving?

_____

_____

_____

_____

_____

4 What is your game plan for week 4? _____

_____

_____

_____

_____

Interact with

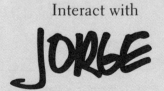

If you would like me to contact you about your progress, send me an e-mail with your answers to this week's update to *weekthree@jorgecruise.com*. I will send you a special e-mail with bonus tips on how to make week 4 even more fun and effective.

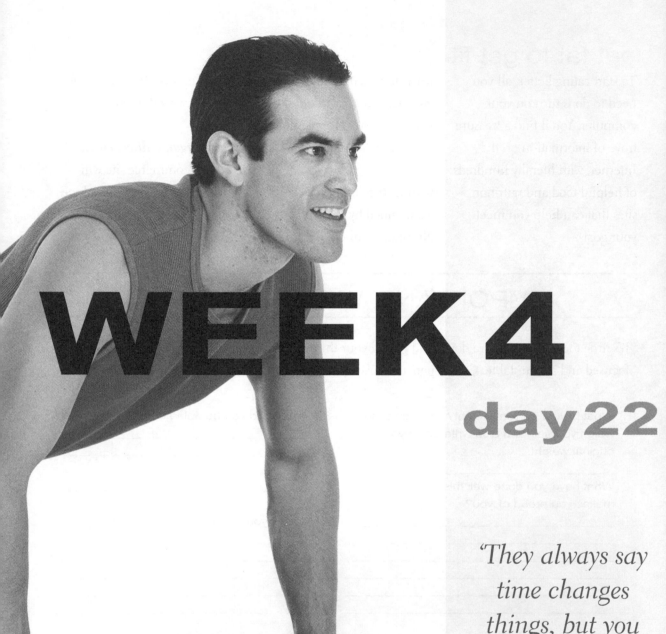

WEEK4
day22

'They always say
time changes
things, but you
actually have to
change them
yourself.'

Andy Warhol
artist

your wake-up talk

The end of your 28-Day Challenge is almost here – just 7 more days to go! This is the day you must strengthen your emotional connection to what you are now doing – exercising and eating well – and what you will continue to do after your official 28-Day Challenge ends.

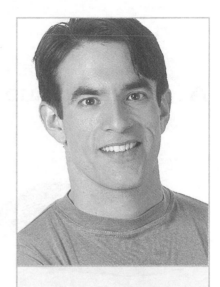

'Recommitting is vital to your success today and forever.'

recommit to your success

Recommitting is vital to your success today . . . and forever. If you are not fully connecting to what you will gain, you will lose your motivation. It's that simple. On the other hand, reminding yourself of your strong Passion Reasons will help you follow through automatically because you will *want to*, not because you have to.

Today, 'raise the bar' another notch by re-reading what you wrote on Week 1 Day 3 (see page 95).

Then I want you to come up with seven more unique benefits that will create more Passion Reasons for continuing with the 8 Minutes in the Morning programme.

7 unique benefits I will gain

1 _____

2 _____

3 _____

4 _____

5 _____

6 _____

7 _____

today's moves
chest and back

EXERCISE LOG					
exercise	lb/kg	set 1 ✓	set 2 ✓	set 3 ✓	set 4 ✓
A					
B					

A chest pushup

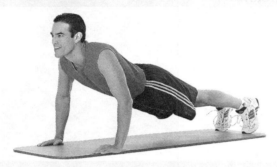 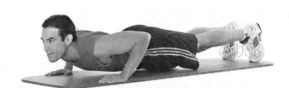

1 On a mat on the floor, start with your arms extended but your elbows slightly bent. Your hands should be slightly wider apart than shoulder-width, and your fingers should be pointing forward. Your toes should be pointing down.

2 Keeping your head up, inhale and slowly bend your elbows as you lower your chest towards the floor. Make sure to keep your back straight and abs tight throughout the move. Stop when your elbows are even with your shoulders. Exhale and slowly raise yourself back to the starting position. If you need to, you can do the easier Knee Pushup on page 116.

eat fat to get fit

Bread is one of the most highly craved carbohydrates, but it doesn't have to be a guilty pleasure.

If you eat wholegrain bread, you'll be consuming slow-release carbohydrates that will keep your insulin levels stable. Be careful when shopping for bread, because the packaging can be misleading.

Just because bread is dark in colour doesn't mean that it contains whole grains. Make sure the label says 'wholemeal', 'wholegrain' or 'wholewheat'. If it says just 'wheat', it may still be refined.

exercise sequence

Warmup
Start your session with a short warmup: jog in place (see page 84).

Training exercises
Do one set of 12 repetitions from exercise A, followed immediately with the same from exercise B. Repeat this cycle for a total of four sets of each exercise, checking them off on your log as you go (see box left).

Cooldown
Finish your session with these three cooldown stretches (see pages 84–5 for full instructions).

Sky-reaching pose: hold for 10 seconds to 1 minute

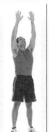

Hurdler's stretch: hold for 10 seconds to 1 minute

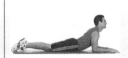

Cobra stretch: hold for 10 seconds to 1 minute

B back superman

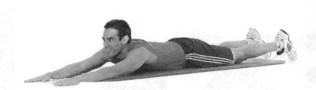 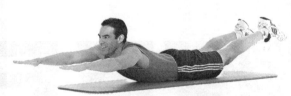

1 Lie on a mat with your belly on the floor, your legs straight and your arms extended in front of you, like Superman flying through the air.

2 Keeping your head up, exhale and simultaneously lift your arms and your legs about 4 in (10 cm) off the ground. If this position puts too much stress on your back, lower your head so that you are looking down at the mat. Hold for 1 second. Inhale while slowly lowering yourself to the starting position.

today's journal

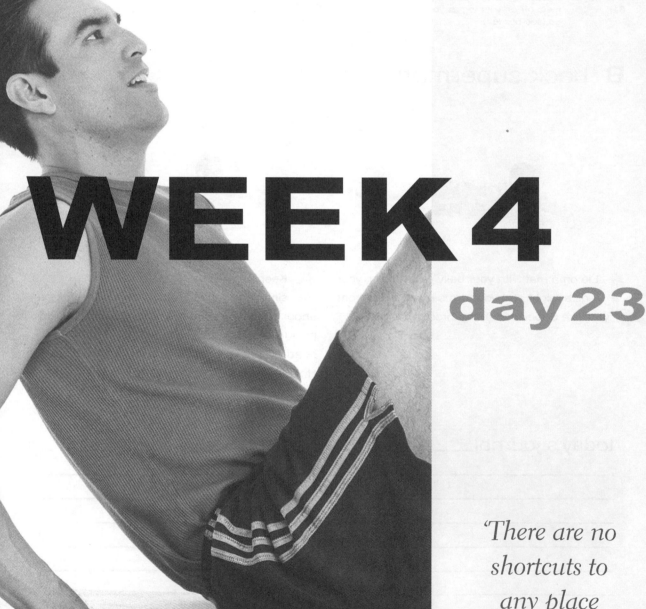

WEEK4
day 23

'There are no
shortcuts to
any place
worth going.'

Source unknown

your wake-up talk

Have you ever looked up to someone? Maybe that someone was a big brother, a big sister, or a good friend – someone who served as a role model to you and who inspired you. A role model can be like a powerful treasure map that shows you the right path. A role model can serve as a blueprint for success and inspiration.

walk your talk

Who will be affected by the new you? Your partner, children, girlfriend, boyfriend, mother, father, best friend, sister, brother, or business associates? Make a list of all the people who will be touched by your new lifestyle. Then briefly write how their lives might change for the better by your being a positive and powerful role model. Get excited!

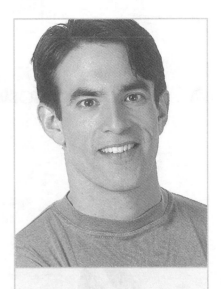

'A role model can serve as a blueprint for success.'

my success inspires others

who: _____ how: _____

who: _____ how: _____

who: _____ how: _____

who: _____ how: _____

who: _____ how: _____

who: _____ how: _____

who: _____ how: _____

who: _____ how: _____

today's moves
shoulders and
abdominals

EXERCISE LOG					
exercise	lb/kg	set 1 ✓	set 2 ✓	set 3 ✓	set 4 ✓
A					
B					

A shoulders forward raise

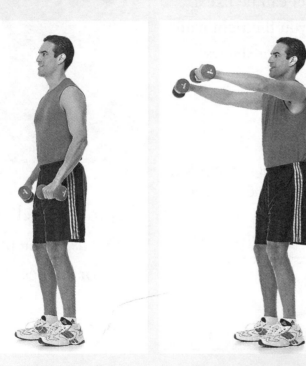

1 Stand with your feet shoulder-width apart. Hold a dumbbell in each hand at your sides.

2 Exhale as you simultaneously raise both arms straight out in front of you. Move only your shoulder joints, keeping your back straight and your elbows slightly bent without being locked. Keep your wrists firm throughout the move. When the dumbbells reach the level of your shoulders, hold for 1 second. Inhale as you lower your hands to the starting position.

eat fat to get fit

Very few people consume all the nutrients they need from food. Even if you eat a healthy diet that is rich in vegetables and whole grains, you may still be deficient in many important nutrients. That's because modern-day farming techniques have depleted some nutrients from the soil, making the foods we eat not as nutritious as they were in the past. To counteract these deficiencies, I suggest that you take a multivitamin every day.

exercise sequence

Warmup
Start your session with a short warmup: jog in place (see page 84).

Training exercises
Do one set of 12 repetitions from exercise A, followed immediately with the same from exercise B. Repeat this cycle for a total of four sets of each exercise, checking them off on your log as you go (see box left).

Cooldown
Finish your session with these three cooldown stretches (see pages 84–5 for full instructions).

Sky-reaching pose: hold for 10 seconds to 1 minute

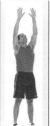

Hurdler's stretch: hold for 10 seconds to 1 minute

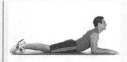

Cobra stretch: hold for 10 seconds to 1 minute

B abdominals lower pull

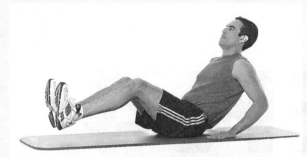

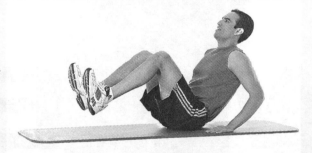

1 Sit on a mat on the floor with your legs slightly bent, your heels just above the floor and your hands behind your buttocks for support.

2 Exhale as you slowly raise your heels and bring your knees towards your torso. When your thighs and abdomen create a 90-degree angle, hold for 1 second. Inhale as you slowly return to the starting position.

today's journal _____ _____

_____ _____

_____ _____

_____ _____

_____ _____

_____ _____

_____ _____

_____ _____

_____ _____

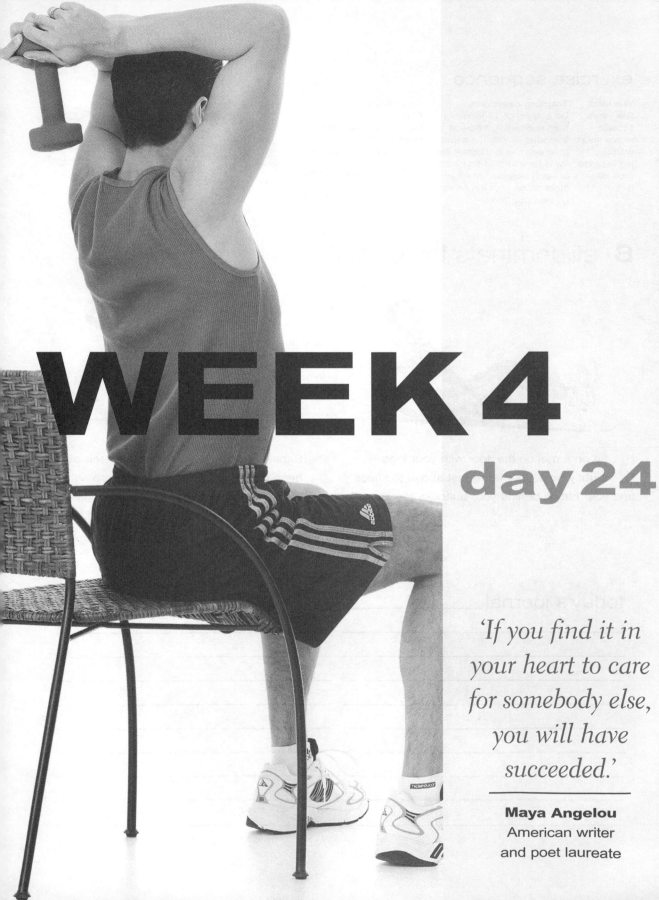

WEEK 4
day 24

'If you find it in your heart to care for somebody else, you will have succeeded.'

Maya Angelou
American writer
and poet laureate

your wake-up talk

You have only 4 days left before your 28-Day Challenge ends – I am so proud of you for coming this far! Do you realize that you are no longer the same person you were when you started this adventure? You have raised your standards and are becoming your very best.

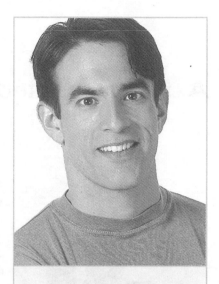

move forward by saying yes

Today's challenge is to embrace the person you have become. Acknowledge all of the transformations that have happened up to this point. Capture all the big and small things that have changed. By recognizing where you are now, you ensure that you will not block further success or revert to the way you were. Write down all of the big and small things that have improved for you. How do you feel and look? How many inches are gone? How is your energy? What clothes fit again? What have people said to you? Pick up a pen and capture everything that is great at the moment.

'Today's challenge is to embrace the person you have become.'

what is great in my life today?

today's moves
triceps and
biceps

EXERCISE LOG					
exercise	lb/kg	set 1 ✓	set 2 ✓	set 3 ✓	set 4 ✓
A					
B					

A triceps seated overhead

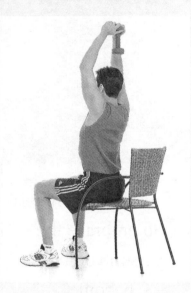

1 Sit in a sturdy chair, grasp a dumbbell with both hands and raise your arms over your head, keeping your elbows slightly bent.

2 Inhale as you slowly bend your elbows and lower the dumbbell behind your head. Keep your elbows as close to your head as possible. When your forearms are parallel to the floor, hold for 1 second. Exhale as you raise the dumbbell to the starting position.

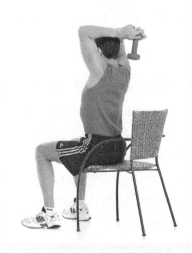

eat fat to get fit

You can increase your chances of following your Eat Fat to Get Fit food plan if you consistently stock your kitchen with the right foods, including whole grains, fresh and frozen vegetables, olive oil, soya products and beans. You can do that by doing a little planning before your shopping excursions.

Never leave the house without a shopping list. Keep your list current by updating it throughout the week as you run out of various foods. Before you leave for the supermarket, do a quick check to see if you need to buy staples such as beans, oils or vegetables. And then eat a small snack. Research shows that people buy more foods that are unhealthy when they shop on empty stomachs. And try not to shop with your children or friends; they may persuade you to buy food that will not support your goals.

exercise sequence

Warmup
Start your session with a short warmup: jog in place (see page 84).

Training exercises
Do one set of 12 repetitions from exercise A, followed immediately with the same from exercise B. Repeat this cycle for a total of four sets of each exercise, checking them off on your log as you go (see box left).

Cooldown
Finish your session with these three cooldown stretches (see pages 84–5 for full instructions).

Sky-reaching pose: hold for 10 seconds to 1 minute

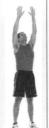

Hurdler's stretch: hold for 10 seconds to 1 minute

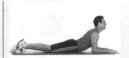

Cobra stretch: hold for 10 seconds to 1 minute

B biceps seated curl

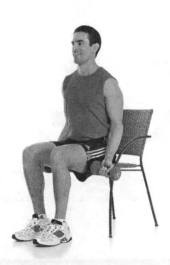

1 Sit on the edge of a sturdy chair and hold a dumbbell in each hand with your arms relaxed at your sides, palms facing out.

2 Exhale as you slowly bend your elbows, curling the dumbbells up towards your shoulders. Keep your wrists straight. When your arms are bent just beyond a 90-degree angle, hold for 1 second. Inhale as you lower the dumbbells to the starting position.

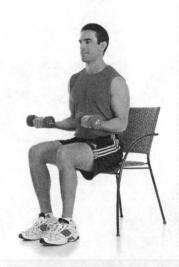

today's journal _____ _____
_____ _____
_____ _____
_____ _____
_____ _____
_____ _____
_____ _____
_____ _____
_____ _____

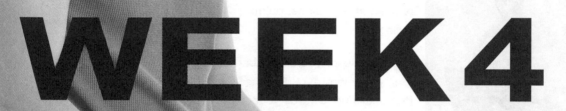

WEEK 4

day 25

'Take heed: you do
not find what you
do not seek.'

English proverb

your wake-up talk

For the next 3 days, I will share resources for you to use to continue your success. Remember that the adventure you have been living for the past month is just the beginning. The best is yet to come!

resources: websites

Today I want to share some valuable websites with you. I have built my whole weight-loss career around the Internet, and I truly believe that it is one of the most powerful tools in today's world. Websites allow us instant access to other people for support, the latest news on health and weight-loss trends, shopping, and great healthy-cooking recipes. Try to visit at least three of my favourite weight-loss websites today. Enjoy!

Check out this list of my favourite websites. Is there a site I missed that you love? E-mail it to *websites@jorgecruise.com*

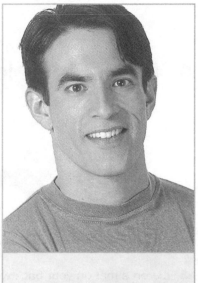

'Try to visit three weight-loss websites today.'

the best weight-loss websites

Eating
www.drweil.com
www.eatright.org
www.prevention.com

Exercise
www.acefitness.org
www.deniseaustin.com
www.ideafit.com

www.kathysmith.com
www.nsmi.org.uk

Motivation
www.ivillage.com
www.miguelruiz.com
www.oprah.com
www.oxygen.com
www.tonyrobbins.com

www.women.com
www.zukav.com

Webcasts (Online TV)
www.changeyourbody.com

Weight-Loss Support
www.jorgecruise.com

today's moves
hamstrings and
quadriceps

EXERCISE LOG					
exercise	lb/kg	set 1 ✓	set 2 ✓	set 3 ✓	set 4 ✓
A					
B					

A hamstrings leg lift

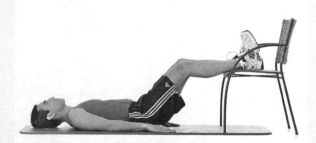 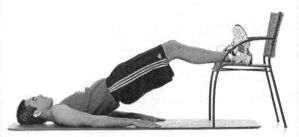

1 Lie on a mat on your back with your palms flat on the mat and your heels on the seat of a sturdy chair.

2 Exhale as you slowly contract the backs of your upper thighs to push your buttocks towards the ceiling. Hold for 1 second. Inhale as you slowly lower your buttocks to the starting point.

eat fat to get fit

On my Eat Fat to Get Fit food plan, you're drinking eight or more glasses of water a day. Try to drink your water at room temperature because water that is too cold can put your body and organs into a state of mild shock. Some people end up with stomach cramps when they drink icy water, especially just after a workout or on a hot day. The contrast between their body temperatures and that of the water is just too great. Room-temperature water is also easier to drink in gulps, making you more likely to fit in those eight glasses.

exercise sequence

Warmup
Start your session with a short warmup: jog in place (see page 84).

Training exercises
Do one set of 12 repetitions from exercise A, followed immediately with one repetition from exercise B. Repeat this cycle for a total of four sets of each exercise, checking them off on your log as you go (see box left).

Cooldown
Finish your session with these three cooldown stretches (see pages 84–5 for full instructions).

Sky-reaching pose: hold for 10 seconds to 1 minute

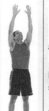

Hurdler's stretch: hold for 10 seconds to 1 minute

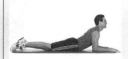
Cobra stretch: hold for 10 seconds to 1 minute

B quadriceps the wall

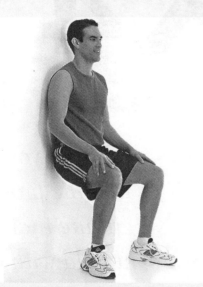

1 Stand with your back against a wall and with your feet shoulder-width apart about 2 ft (60 cm) in front of the wall. Rest your hands on your thighs. Slowly slide down the wall, bending your knees until you are in a high seated position. Hold for 1 minute, making sure to breathe deeply while holding. *Do only one repetition for this exercise.*

today's journal

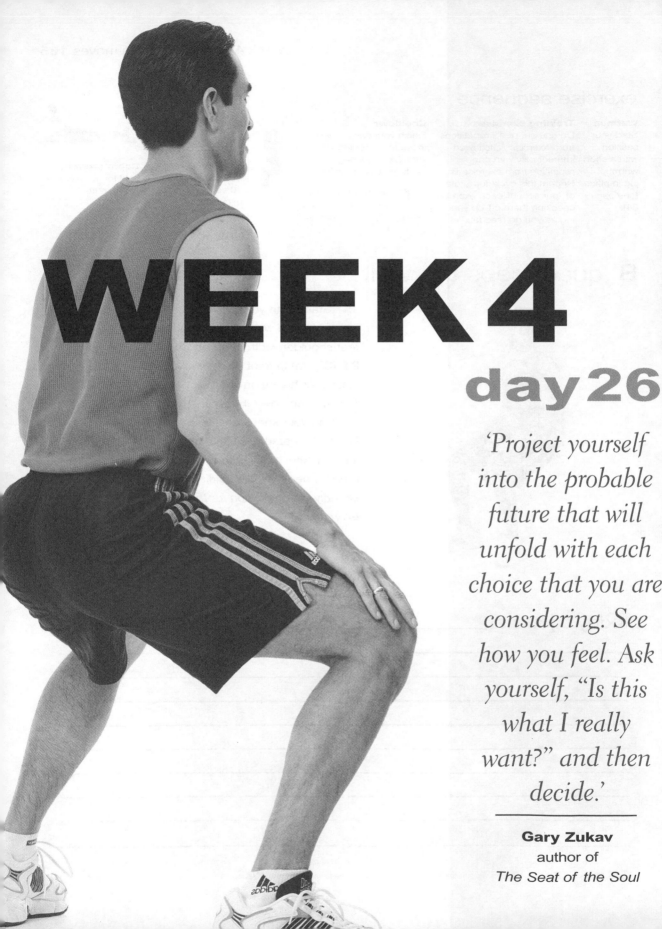

WEEK 4

day 26

'Project yourself into the probable future that will unfold with each choice that you are considering. See how you feel. Ask yourself, "Is this what I really want?" and then decide.'

Gary Zukav
author of
The Seat of the Soul

your wake-up talk

A magazine subscription is one of the best gifts you can give yourself and others because it is like having a good friend with great ideas and inspirational photos turn up on your doorstep.

resources: magazines

It's a wonderful advantage to have an automatic source of inspiration and information enter your world consistently. It sets you up to win! When you least expect it or remember it, there it is in your letter box.

Today, check out some of the best magazines at the newsagents or in a bookshop. Flip through them. Eventually, I want you to subscribe to one of these magazines for monthly inspiration.

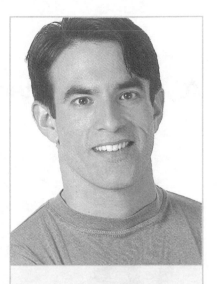

'Today, check out some of the best health magazines.'

the best magazines

Do you have a favourite magazine that isn't on the list? E-mail your suggestion to *magazines@jorgecruise.com*.

Good Health	Shape
Health & Fitness	Slimmer, Healthier, Fitter
Men's Health	Top Santé
Natural Health & Wellbeing	Women's Health
O, The Oprah Magazine	Zest

To receive your copy of the 8 Minutes in the Morning newsletter, visit my website at *www.jorgecruise.com*.

today's moves
calves and
buttocks

EXERCISE LOG					
exercise	lb/kg	set 1 ✓	set 2 ✓	set 3 ✓	set 4 ✓
A					
B					

A calves seated raise

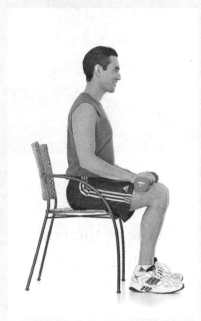

1 Sit in a sturdy chair with your feet flat on the floor and hold a dumbbell in place on top of each knee.

2 Exhale as you slowly lift your heels, keeping your toes on the floor. You should feel this in your calves. Hold for 1 second. Inhale as you lower your heels to the starting position.

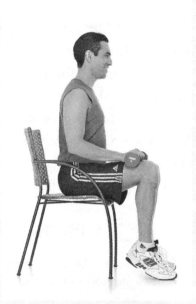

eat fat to get fit

There's nothing like a cold or the flu to derail your best fitness intentions. Yes, you should rest while you're sick. But taking a few days off can get you out of your exercise habit, so try to stay as healthy as possible.

One way you can ward off a cold or the flu is by eating lots of garlic. It's a natural germ fighter and immunity booster, especially when you eat it raw.

Try crushing a few cloves, placing them on a spoon

and swallowing them. Follow it with a sip of water. Crushing the garlic means that you don't have to chew it in your mouth and get that garlicky smell on your breath.

exercise sequence

Warmup
Start your session with a short warmup: jog in place (see page 84).

Training exercises
Do one set of 12 repetitions from exercise A, followed immediately with the same from exercise B. Repeat this cycle for a total of four sets of each exercise, checking them off on your log as you go (see box left).

Cooldown
Finish your session with these three cooldown stretches (see pages 84–5 for full instructions).

Sky-reaching pose: hold for 10 seconds to 1 minute

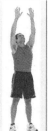

Hurdler's stretch: hold for 10 seconds to 1 minute

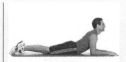

Cobra stretch: hold for 10 seconds to 1 minute

B buttocks wide squeeze

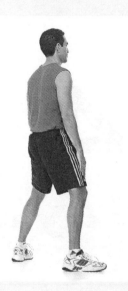

1 Stand with your feet slightly wider than shoulder-width apart, your arms at your sides and your knees slightly bent.

2 Inhale as you bend your knees to 90 degrees, making sure to squeeze your buttock muscles. Hold for 1 second. Exhale as you slowly push through your buttocks back to the starting position.

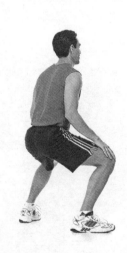

today's journal _____ _____

_____ _____

_____ _____

_____ _____

_____ _____

_____ _____

_____ _____

_____ _____

_____ _____

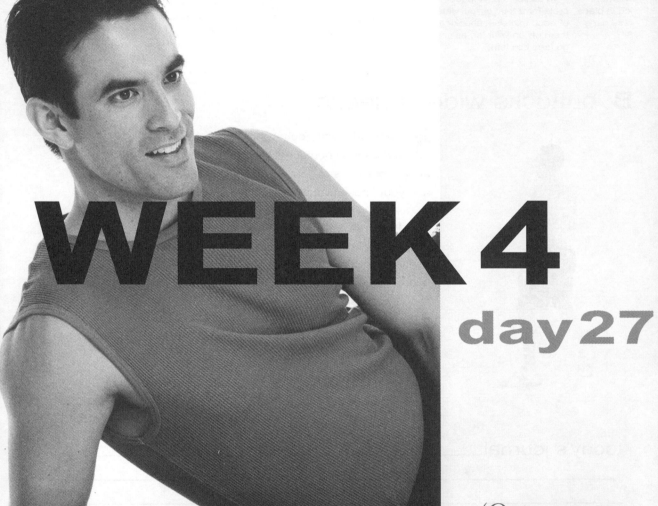

WEEK 4

day 27

'One can never
consent to creep
when one feels an
impulse to soar.'

Helen Keller
writer and social
reformer

your wake-up talk

Books are great resources, and with all the wonderful information, inspiration and guidance you can find inside, they are sometimes like a best friend. Books have the power to change your life, as they are often the product of many years of study and experience from experts passionate about their messages.

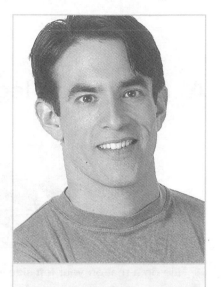

resources: reference books

I have many favourite books on my bookshelf. I recommend that, like me, you add as many as possible to your weight-loss library. How essential is a good book? I keep a quote in my office from Erasmus, one of the greatest scholars of all time, who lived during the Renaissance: 'When I get a little money, I buy books; and if any is left, I buy food and clothes.'

'Books have the power to change your life.'

the best weight-loss reference books

You can order any of these books online or from your favourite bookshop.

As a Man Thinketh by James Allen

Awaken the Giant Within by Anthony Robbins

Banish Your Belly, Butt and Thighs by the editors of *Prevention* Health Books for Women

Dr Shapiro's Picture Perfect Weight Loss by Howard M Shapiro

Eat Fat, Lose Weight by Ann Louise Gittleman, MS, CSN

Eating Well for Optimum Health by Andrew Weil, MD

Get a Real Food Life by Janine Whiteson

100 Ways to Motivate Yourself by Steve Chandler

Powerfully Fit by Brian Chichester, Jack Croft and the editors of *Men's Health books*

Revitalize Your Life by Jack LaLanne

Strong Women Stay Slim by Miriam E. Nelson

Think and Grow Rich by Napoleon Hill

Weight Training for Dummies by Liz Neporent and Suzanne Schlosberg

Win the Fat War by Anne Alexander

Workouts for Dummies by Tamilee Webb

today's moves
inner thigh and
outer thigh

EXERCISE LOG					
exercise	lb/kg	set 1 ✓	set 2 ✓	set 3 ✓	set 4 ✓
A					
B					

A inner thigh leg raise

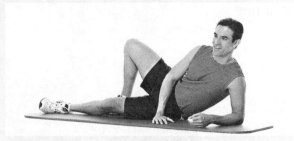 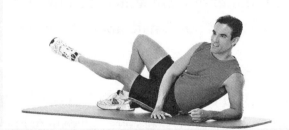

1 Lie on a mat on your left side with your left elbow and forearm supporting your upper body and your left leg extended. Bend your right knee and place your right foot behind your left leg for balance.

2 Keeping your left leg straight, exhale as you slowly lift your left foot as high as you can. Hold for 1 second. Inhale as you lower your foot to the starting position. Do one set with your left leg, then switch sides.

eat fat to get fit

In keeping with today's 'book' theme, I want to recommend *Diet for a New America* by John Robbins.

After I read this book, I never looked at food the same way again. It will help you in your journey to Eat Fat to Get Fit, and I promise that it will give you a powerful advantage in your long-term weight loss.

Dr Andrew Weil, highly regarded by me and millions of others, has stated that: '*Diet for a New America* should be read by everyone interested in healthy living. It is a well-researched, well-documented and eye-opening account of the myths and truths about meat, milk, fat and protein.

'I will recommend this book to patients, friends and relatives.'

exercise sequence

Warmup
Start your session with a short warmup: jog in place (see page 84).

Training exercises
Do one set of 12 repetitions from exercise A, followed immediately with the same from exercise B. Repeat this cycle for a total of four sets of each exercise, checking them off on your log as you go (see box left).

Cooldown
Finish your session with these three cooldown stretches (see pages 84–5 for full instructions).

Sky-reaching pose: hold for 10 seconds to 1 minute

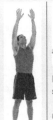

Hurdler's stretch: hold for 10 seconds to 1 minute

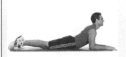

Cobra stretch: hold for 10 seconds to 1 minute

B outer thigh leg raise

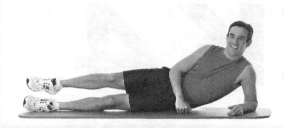

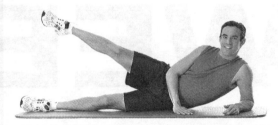

1 Lie on a mat on your left side. Support your upper body with your left elbow. Your legs should be extended and aligned with your upper body.

2 Exhale as you slowly raise your upper leg. Hold for 1 second. Inhale as you slowly lower your leg to the starting position. Repeat 12 times with your left leg, then switch sides. For more resistance, wear ankle weights.

today's journal _____

WEEK4
day28

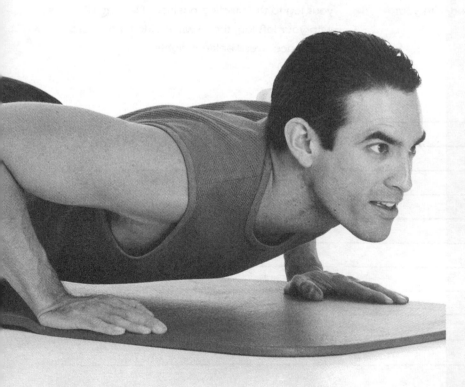

'Nothing splendid
has ever been
achieved except by
those who believed
that something
inside of them
was superior to
circumstance.'

Bruce Barton
advertising executive, writer
and congressman

your wake-up talk

You've finished, right? Well, not exactly. You have been living a new lifestyle for 28 days. You now have a 'lean machine' in place or are well on your way. But you must continue to move forward. By raising your standards, you are a new person. What once felt good will no longer feel the same.

celebrate

Imagine that you had never learned to walk and can only crawl. It would cause back problems and hurt your knees. You wake up every morning with a sore back and a feeling of fatigue. Now imagine that you have finally learned to walk. The pain and discomfort disappear. Why in the world would you go back to crawling on your knees? That's exactly how you must think.

Now that you have crossed the first 28-day finish line, celebrate and continue to move forwards. Depending on how much more fat you need to burn, follow the 28-Day Challenge for another cycle. Each time you do, you will become healthier and fitter and feel better and better, guaranteed!

Grab a pen and write down exactly what you are going to do to commit yourself to living this new lifestyle.

This is your day off, so take some extra time for yourself. Go for a powerwalk, get some fresh air, and keep motivating yourself.

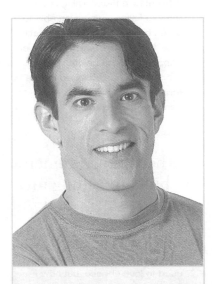

'Celebrate and continue to move forwards.'

what will I do to continue?

E-mail your success story and photo to *photo@jorgecruise.com*. I look forward to hearing from you.

_____

_____

_____

_____

_____

8 minute marvel Lisa lost 20 lbs (10 kg)!

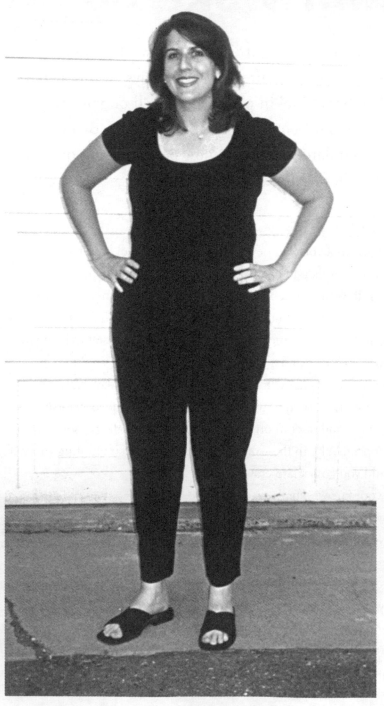

8 Minutes in the Morning is so easy to follow. I was even able to go on holiday for a week and still lose 1 lb (0.5kg), which has never happened to me before. This programme has changed my life in more ways than one. I love the personal development.

'I am not only becoming thinner but also getting my self-esteem back.'

And the Eat Fat to Get Fit food plan is now a way of life for me. I used to love cheese, but now I don't even crave it. I have tons of energy and am very excited at my progress.

Lisa DelVaglio
Sales Representative

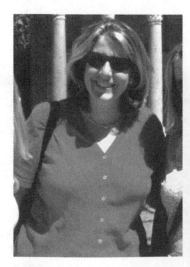

before

eat fat to get fit

I'm not a big fan of salt – and neither are most doctors. Besides being connected with high blood pressure, salt also makes you retain water. So when you gain several pounds, it may well be from water, not fat.

Instead of seasoning your food with salt, try fresh herbs such as basil, coriander and oregano. Remember that cooking and eating are an *adventure*. Expand your tastes beyond salt and discover a whole new world of eating.

IMPORTANT: WEEK 4 UPDATE

Congratulations! You did it! Now it's time to monitor how well you are doing and record your fourth week's progress. This will keep you focused and accountable. Grab a pen and answer the following questions.

1 What is your current weight? Use scales to weigh yourself and also write down your original weight. _____

2 What have you done well this week? What makes you proud of you?

_____
_____
_____
_____
_____
_____

3 What could you be doing better or improving?

_____
_____
_____

4 What is your game plan for week 5 and beyond?

_____
_____
_____

When you have finished, have your 'after' photo taken, then tape it next to your 'before' photo on page 39.

Interact with

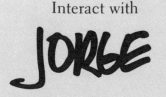

If you would like to get more interactive, e-mail the answers for this week's update to *weekfour@jorgecruise.com*. I will send you a special e-mail with bonus tips on how to maintain and even further your success. Include your story, how much weight you have lost, how your life has changed and what you are most excited and proud about.

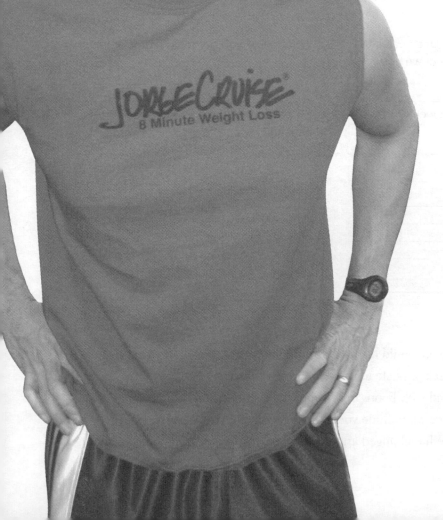

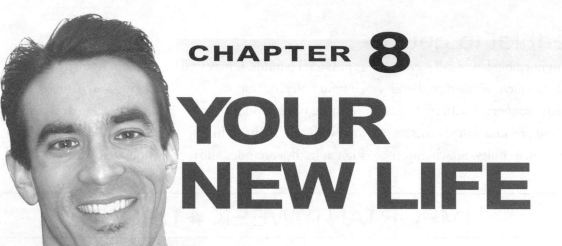

CHAPTER **8**
YOUR
NEW LIFE

how to maintain your success or lose more weight

You have just completed my 8 Minutes in the Morning weight-loss programme. Well done, and congratulations on your success!

savour your success

In my introduction, I told you that you would get hooked on this way of living. Remember how I compared your old lifestyle to crawling and your new lifestyle to walking? Now that you can walk, why would you go back to crawling? You've invested your energy and effort in making better choices that have helped you lose weight. You made choices that will keep you feeling and looking great forever. Keep up the good work!

So what do you do now? Whether you've arrived at your weight-loss goal or not, sticking with the programme is the number one way to look and feel your best. If you still have weight to lose, simply restart the 4-week transformation cycle.

Each time you go through this cycle, you'll get better and better results and that will ensure your long-term success.

But before you move on, I want you to savour your current success. Read back over your journal entries from the past 28 days. Relish how much you've changed and how far you have come. You have grown fit from the inside out. Treat yourself to the reward you wrote down on

keep the weight off

To continue the success of my 8 Minutes in the Morning programme, follow these simple new rules:

1 If you want to keep the weight off or lose even more, you have to keep doing your

your questions

When I do the leg lifts in your programme, I don't feel like I'm working hard any more. Is something wrong?

You've become stronger and your body weight is no longer heavy enough. Congratulations! To make these exercises more effective now, invest in some ankle weights with Velcro straps. I like the kind that comes with removable weights so you can continue to add weight as your body grows stronger.

Week 2 Day 13 (see page 135). Now's the time to take that mini-vacation, buy a new outfit, or spend a day at the spa . . . you've earned it!

8 Minutes in the Morning workouts. Repeat the same exercise routine as you did for weeks 1 to 4, but *increase the amount of weight you are lifting*. This is critical! Remember that muscle gets

stronger only if you push it beyond what is comfortable. And the more lean tissue you have, the higher your metabolism will be.

2 As you lose weight, switch to the calorie selection that is appropriate for your new weight. The Eating Card System will help keep you honest, so use it.

3 Get on the scales to monitor your weight loss every Sunday. If you start regaining weight, jump to the Quick Start selection and follow it diligently to get back on track.

4 No matter what happens, never skip meals. Eat at least 3 meals a day, and always have fat with each meal. If you miss a meal, you are more likely to overeat at night. If you get hungry, snack on the unlimited vegetables (see page 220).

5 Review Your Wake-Up Talks. Your motivation needs to be exercised daily, too.

6 Remember that setbacks are only challenges in disguise. Look at them as lessons. If you eat more than you should or you miss a day of exercise,

don't waste time beating yourself up. Just get back on track and focus on what you want. It's up to you, and you will do it!

your questions

What do you think of alternative methods of exercise such as yoga and tai chi?

While they are not the most effective types of exercises for weight loss, these disciplines are excellent for variety and stress reduction. They will help focus your mind and spirit on inner tranquillity and peace.

share your success:
the only way to enjoy weight loss

Probably the most valuable lesson I have learned from my 3 million weight-loss clients is that the way to truly enjoy weight loss and maintain your success is to share it with someone else. Giving someone else what you have discovered is one of the greatest joys in life. It's a privilege (and addictive!) to help others take charge of their lives and happiness.

My clients who lost weight and then helped someone else do the same are just as motivated

months and years later as they were on Day 1. When you share your success, everyone wins.

In that spirit, I'd like to share the success story from one of my first clients, Joe Newsome. Joe lost 2 st 12 lb (18 kg) with 8 Minutes in the Morning and then went on to help transform his family, friends and colleagues. Here is his inspiring story:

'I've witnessed an incredible change in my life, a change that is so wonderful and is available

to anyone who wants to become lean, healthy and happy about themselves.

'I'm 5 ft 7 in (1.7 m) tall, and before I discovered Jorge's 8 Minutes in the Morning programme, I weighed 14 st 6 lb (92 kg). I would trudge up the stairs to my house and feel winded. I hurt whenever I tried to run and play with my sons. I lacked the energy to get out of bed in the morning.

'A family history of heart disease scared me, and I finally

8 minute marvel Joe lost 40 lbs (18 kg)!

A family history of heart disease scared me, and I finally decided that I would try to lose the weight.

I started the programme and saw results within the first week: I began sleeping better, my energy increased, my weight dropped and I felt better about myself. The benefits just kept coming. My body began to start shaping up, the swelling in my feet disappeared, the pain in my joints began to subside and I even stopped snoring. Best of all, I felt as if I had moved from my mid-thirties back into my twenties!

'All of the knowledge I needed to lose the weight was packed into one book and laid out for me on a daily basis.'

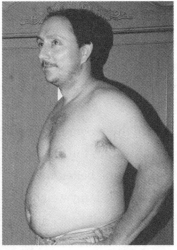

before

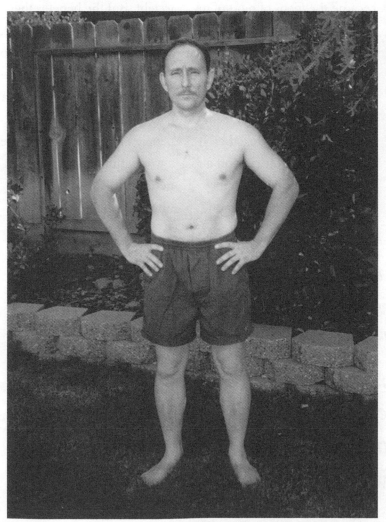

after
Joe now feels good enough about his body to garden without his shirt on!

decided that I would try to lose the weight, so I began my search for help on the Internet. I came across Jorge's website and liked what I saw. His programme didn't include pills or chemicals. Instead, it focused on building muscle and eating the right kinds of foods and fats. All of the knowledge I needed to lose the weight was packed into one book and laid out for me on a daily basis.

'I started the programme and saw results within the first week: I began sleeping better, my energy increased, my weight dropped and I felt better about myself. The benefits just kept coming. My body began to start shaping up, the swelling in my feet disappeared, the pain in my joints began to subside and I even stopped snoring. Best of all, I felt as if I had moved from my mid-thirties back into my twenties!

'My friends, family and colleagues soon began asking me about what I was doing. Answering questions about 8 Minutes in the Morning soon became the focus of most of my conversations. The interest grew so large that I decided to form an 8 Minutes in the Morning team.

'I created a sign-up sheet and, 22 names later, we were ready to kick off our 28 days together. It was awesome as the support and inspiration continued to grow. Each pound lost was everyone's gain. Recipes, ideas and tips were passed around through e-mail, and everybody inspired each other. We were one proud team!

'Sharing this programme was an incredible blessing. I was attempting to pay back my friends and colleagues for all of the inspiration that they had given me while I was losing weight. But the benefits they achieved left me feeling so great and helped me grow even more with the programme. It is one of the best feelings to share such a great change. Sharing in people's health and giving them a wonderful opportunity for a new, healthy lifestyle is the ultimate gift.'

'Sharing this programme was an incredible blessing. I was attempting to pay back my friends and colleagues for all of the inspiration that they had given me while I was losing weight. But the benefits they achieved left me feeling so great and helped me grow even more with the programme.'

my dream

In the Emotional Advantage chapter, I shared with you the power of having a specific goal. Well, it is my goal and greatest hope to be able to reach as many new people as I have already coached online. I want to change the lives of at least another 3 million people with this book. Remember that every 5 minutes, 3 people die in the United States due to problems related to obesity. And I can only do this with your support and success. By working together as a team, we can do this, and we will succeed – one person at a time!

What can you do to help make a big difference? Log on to *www.jorgecruise.com/share* and send a quick, but life-changing e-mail to all your friends about 8 Minutes in the Morning. But regardless, please do keep in touch with me directly at *coach@jorgecruise.com* and visit me at my website, *jorgecruise.com*, too. Send me your story and your 'before' and 'after' photos. Tell your friends and family about your success with the 8 Minutes in the Morning programme, and before you know it, a worldwide revolution will be under way.

Above all, thanks for allowing me to be your coach on your amazing weight-loss adventure. I wish you the best. I know you will do it!

POWER-WALKING

exercising your heart

Though strength training is the smarter way to lose weight, you need to do some form of aerobic exercise to truly condition your heart and lungs. And compared to all other forms of aerobic exercise, walking is the most convenient way to get your heart rate pumping. That's why walking goes hand in hand with the core 8 Minutes in the Morning programme.

'Walking will strengthen your heart and decrease your risk of disease.'

the benefits of walking

My powerwalking plan will help you tap into 'quick bonus' calories. Each time you walk for at least 20 minutes, you'll burn an average of 150 to 200 additional calories. If you walk 6 times per week at lunchtime or as an evening break, that could add up to 1,200 weekly calories, which adds up to an additional ½ lb (250g) of fat per week, or *an extra 2 lb (1 kg)* of fat per month. The bottom line is that adding powerwalking to your programme will help you meet your weight-loss goals even faster.

So here is what I recommend: always do the strength training in the morning because it is the most effective weight-loss solution, and fit in aerobic exercise when you have more time, want to burn more calories and, just as important, want to keep your heart and lungs strong.

Too often people who have a significant amount of weight to lose start aerobic exercise without first getting strong. Extra fat coupled with weak muscles makes aerobic exercise feel more taxing than it should. Your thighs might rub together and chafe; your joints may hurt under the weight of your body; you may simply have a tough time moving. Also, I hear from

plenty of women and men who are too embarrassed to exercise at the gym in front of all of those hard bodies.

My 8 Minutes in the Morning powerwalking programme addresses all of those concerns. After just 1 week of my 8 Minutes in the Morning programme, many of these concerns will subside. Remember that my programme not only helps you firm up from the outside but from the inside as well. That means you'll find confidence that you didn't know you had. And eventually, those fears of exercising in public will subside.

There are many reasons walking is extremely good for you. It will strengthen your heart and decrease your risk of various diseases, from heart disease to cancer to diabetes. Walking also helps when you're mad, sad, can't think straight or when your mood is making you think about food.

The combination of getting your heart rate up and spending time outdoors melts stress away, making you more effective in everything you do. A 30-minute powerwalk leaves you relaxed and rejuvenated.

How many times have you decided not to do something or put your life on hold because you couldn't keep up or were too out of shape? Maybe your kids wanted to explore a nature trail or go to a theme park, and you weren't sure if you were up to it. Maybe a friend wanted to go on an all-day shopping spree in town, or your partner suggested a romantic stroll on the pier. My powerwalking plan will help you get in shape so that you will never have to use your body as an excuse again.

Studies show that most people who start powerwalking stick with it, compared to only half of those who try swimming, stair-stepping or other forms of aerobic activity. That's probably because walking is one of the easiest activities to fit into a busy day. (You can do it anywhere – even when you go on holiday.)

Walking outside also gets you in touch with nature. The wind, fresh air, sunlight, natural colours and animal life can all invigorate you. If you're walking in the early morning or in the evening when it's dark, wear

work powerwalking into your day

Walking makes for a great break from your workday. Go for a walk in your lunch break to burn off stress, or do it after work to settle into the evening. To encourage yourself, and to get the most out of your powerwalking experience, try the following:

- Walk with your family after work, using the time to catch up and spend quality time together.
- Walk with colleagues, instead of congregating in the canteen.
- Walk any time someone gets on your nerves. It will help you rid your brain of those negative thoughts so that you can return to work focused.
- Walk every chance you get, even if that means parking in the space furthest from the supermarket, doing laps around your doctor's office as you wait for your appointment, or taking a quick stroll as dinner cooks in the oven.
- Walk with a friend instead of going out to eat or chatting on the phone.
- Schedule your powerwalks on your calendar.
- Think of walking as time to yourself away from life's other hassles.
- Get others involved. You'll be amazed at how far and how fast you can go when you have a juicy conversation to fuel the walk.
- Walk to a destination. Go on an 'errand walk' where you get money from the cashpoint, pick up supplies from the DIY shop, or return a borrowed book to a friend.
- Notice your surroundings. Try to recognize the birds you see, or the trees and plants that you pass. If you're in a city, enjoy the window displays.
- Get a dog. Your dog just won't let you get out of it.

light-coloured, reflective clothing to make yourself visible to oncoming cars. Carry a small torch in each hand. Attach cheap reflective tape to your clothes, or buy a reflective vest. And whenever you walk in the dark, try to do it with a companion. If the weather makes walking outdoors uncomfortable, or if safety is an issue, move indoors. Walk at a shopping centre or other large building. You can powerwalk through a supermarket, or even up and down hallways in a hotel. Investing in a treadmill for your home gym is a great way to make sure you can exercise every day.

your questions

I'd like to try powerwalking, but I'm too self-conscious to let my friends and neighbours see me. How do I get over my fear?

If you feel embarrassed about walking or doing other fitness activities in public, 8 Minutes in the Morning can help. As you progress through the programme, your confidence will grow with each Wake-Up Talk. And as you lose weight, it will become that much easier to feel good about yourself. Remember, you need to focus on what you are doing for yourself, not on what others might think.

what to wear for powerwalking

The most important gear you need for walking is a sturdy pair of walking shoes. Those flimsy flats, loafers or pumps that you wear to work simply aren't right for powerwalking. They'll slow you down, make you feel off-balance and may make your legs ache. Even if you powerwalk in your work clothes, I suggest that you put on a pair of trainers. You need good arch support and lots of cushioning. The more you weigh, the more support you'll need.

You can buy your trainers at a department store or a sports shop. They don't have to cost a lot of money, but they should fit well and feel good. It's best to try them on in the afternoon, since your feet tend to swell during the day. Walk around the shop and concentrate on how they feel. Does your heel slide up and down in the shoe? If so, you'll end up getting blisters. Do your toes feel pinched? Just imagine how they'll feel after 20 minutes of powerwalking.

Replace your shoes about every 6 months, or sooner. Pay attention to how your feet feel when you walk. As soon as they start to feel sore, replace your shoes. Also, your feet may shrink as you lose weight, which means that you'll need a new pair.

In addition to trainers, you can buy an array of synthetic clothing that will soak up moisture away from your body, keeping you dry and comfortable in both hot and cold weather. In the summer, light tops made of CoolMax and other synthetic materials keep you cool and dry and feel much lighter than cotton or any other natural fibre. In the winter, multiple layers of synthetic tights, long-sleeved shirts and jackets will block out the wind and keep you toasty without making you feel bulky.

how far, how fast?

When you first start walking, you might only be able to make it to the end of your driveway or to the end of your block. That's fine. You're out there and you're trying. And you just walked more than you walked yesterday. So give yourself a big pat on the back. After all, 1 minute or 5 minutes is better than no minutes at all.

For your first walk, go until you run out of breath or you start to tire. Build from there, increasing your time about 10 per cent each week. Eventually, you want to be able to walk for 26 continuous minutes. (If you end up getting hooked and going much longer than 26 minutes, good for you! But I'm only asking you to do 26 minutes.) Three of those minutes should be a jog-in-place warmup (see page 84) and 3 of them the cooldown stretches on the page opposite. If you skip either of these, you risk injury. The warmup gets the fluid in your joints ready for the faster walking; the cooldown helps blood flow back to your heart instead of pooling in your legs, making you feel faint and weak.

Work on your distance first, then your intensity. You shouldn't pant and your legs shouldn't hurt. If you feel either, you're walking too fast or too far for your fitness level. Back off a little and then slowly add distance or intensity. If you rate your effort on a scale from 1 to 10, it should fall somewhere between 6 and 8. That's your fat-burning zone. You'll feel better in that zone as well as reap the most benefits from the exercise.

how to powerwalk well

Powerwalking with proper posture will save your knees, especially if you still have a lot of weight to lose.

Walking with good form will also increase the number of calories you burn and make your walk more enjoyable. You want walking to be a *total-body experience*, not just something that involves your legs, so make an effort to use your upper body, which will increase your caloric burn.

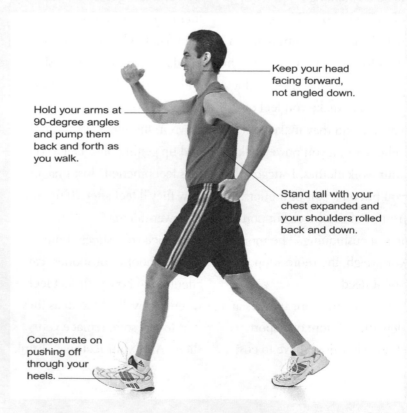

Keep your head facing forward, not angled down.

Hold your arms at 90-degree angles and pump them back and forth as you walk.

Stand tall with your chest expanded and your shoulders rolled back and down.

Concentrate on pushing off through your heels.

AFTER-WALK STRETCHES

I recommend that you do the following stretches. It's always best to stretch after your walk, when the muscles are already warm.

Calf Stretch: Stand 2 to 3 ft (60 to 90 cm) away from a wall. Place your palms on the wall with your left foot in front of the other, about 2 ft (60 cm) apart. Lean into the wall with your left leg bent and your right leg straight. Feel the stretch in your calf. Hold for 20 seconds and then switch legs.

Deep Calf Stretch: Stand 2 to 3ft (60 to 90 cm) away from a wall. Place your palms on the wall with your left foot in front of the other, about 2 ft (60 cm) apart. Lean into the wall with your left leg bent and your right leg straight, then bend your right leg so that the stretch moves to a different area on your calf. Hold for 20 seconds and then switch legs.

Hamstring Stretch: Lie on your back on a mat with your legs bent. Bring your left leg up and thread a towel around your thigh. Hold your thigh at about a 90-degree angle (if you can). Straighten your leg as much as possible. Hold for 20 seconds and then switch legs.

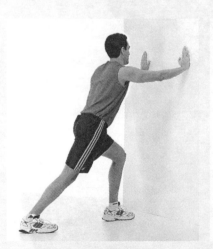
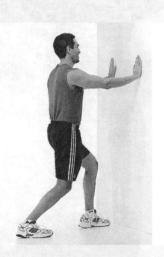
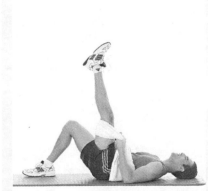

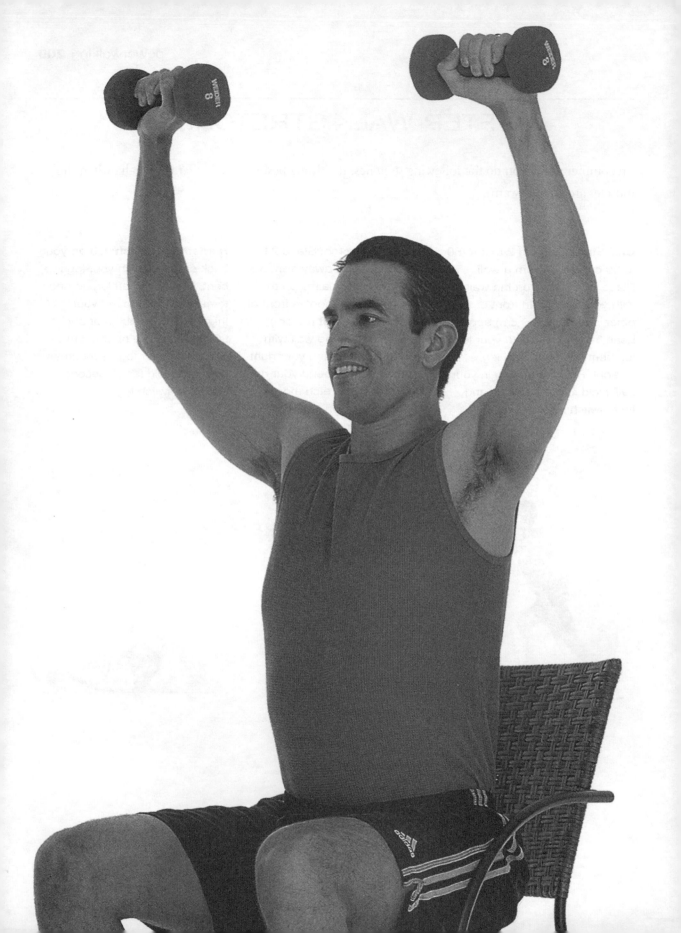

4
Resources

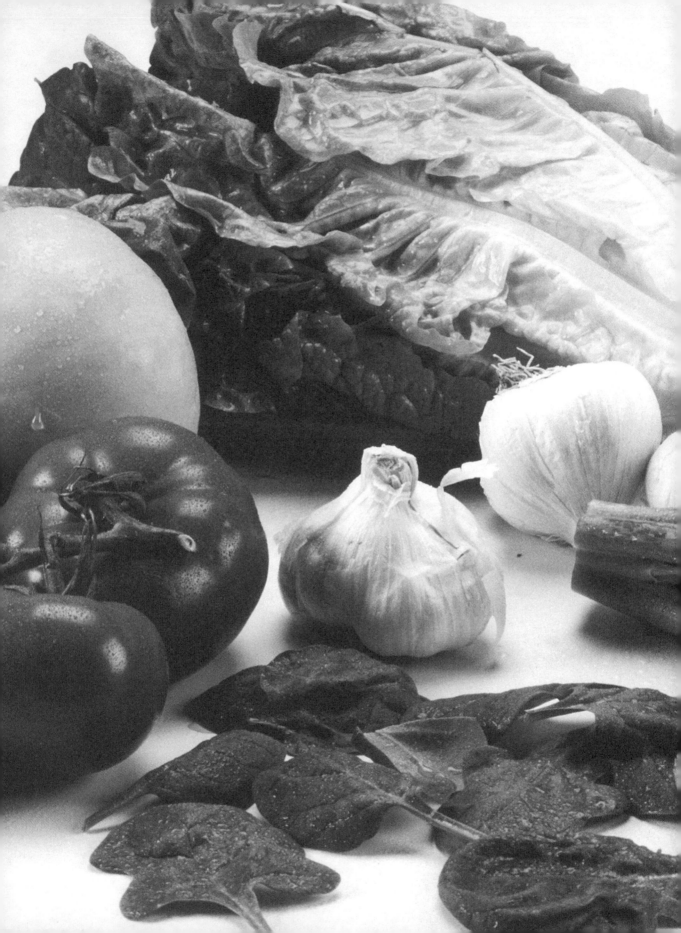

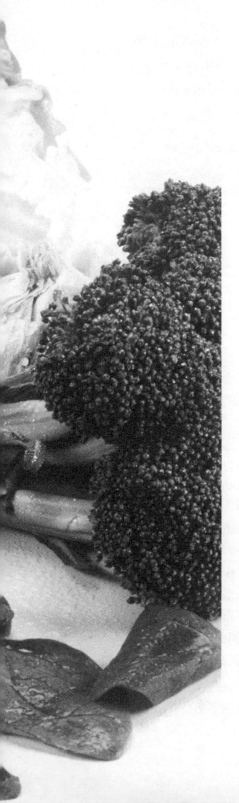

the easy way to eat fat to get fit

The following pages will be invaluable to you as you begin and maintain the 8 Minutes in the Morning way of life. Use these pages for quick reference and to guide your daily food choices. Everything's here:

- A comprehensive **Food List**, showing how much food equals one box on your Eating Card
- Exciting and simple-to-make recipes to help you get those veggies into your meals effortlessly
- The very important **quick start menu plan**, which makes your first week of eating healthier a 'no-brainer'
- **The Eating Cards**, your insurance policy for eating right every day

There are two blank Eating Cards on page 235 for you to copy, cut out, staple together and carry with you. Make four copies to get enough cards for a week, plus one extra. Give the extra to a friend and introduce her to a new 8 Minutes in the Morning life, too!

food list

Here is everything you need to know about the foods you can eat and the proper serving sizes. This is what each box on your Eating Card equals. These (approximate) caloric values have been developed by the American Dietetic Association.

Fat = 45 calories
Dairy foods = 90 calories
Protein = 75 calories
Complex Carbohydrate = 80 calories

Vegetables = 25 calories
Fruit = 60 calories
Treats and cravings = 30 calories

fat

Unless otherwise specified, cross off 1 Fat box on your Eating Card for each specified amount.

Preferred fats

Almond butter, 1 tablespoon –
    PLUS 1 Protein box
Almonds, raw, 6
Avocado, ⅛ medium
Cashews, 6
Flax oil, 1 teaspoon or 4 capsules
Oil-based salad dressing, 1 tablespoon
Olive oil, 1 teaspoon
Olives, 10 small or 5 large
Peanut butter, 2 teaspoons – PLUS 1 Protein box
Peanuts, 10
Pecans, 4 halves
Pumpkin seeds, 1 tablespoon
Sesame seeds, 1 tablespoon
Soya mayonnaise, 1 tablespoon
Sunflower seeds, 1 tablespoon
Tahini paste, 2 teaspoons

Fats to minimize

Butter, reduced-calorie,
    1 tablespoon
Butter, 1 teaspoon
Coconut, 2 tablespoons
Corn oil, 1 teaspoon
Cream cheese, 1 tablespoon
Cream cheese, reduced-calorie, 2 tablespoons
Lard, 1 teaspoon
Mayonnaise, 1 teaspoon
Mayonnaise, reduced-calorie, 1 tablespoon
Single cream, 2 tablespoons
Sour cream, 2 tablespoons
Sour cream, reduced-calorie, 3 tablespoons
Vegetable cooking fat, 1 teaspoon

dairy foods

For portions of cheese that have up to 320 calories per 100g, cross off 1 Dairy and 1 Fat box per ounce unless otherwise specified. For cheese portions that are whole-milk varieties (more than 320 calories per 100g), cross off 1 Dairy and 2 Fat boxes unless otherwise specified.

Cheese (less than 320 per 100 g)

Cottage, low-fat or fat-free, 4 tablespoons
Ricotta, low-fat or fat-free, 4 tablespoons
Soya, all varieties, 1 oz (30 g)

Cheese (more than 320 calories per 100 g)

Brie, 1 oz (30 g)
Cheddar, 1 oz (30 g)
Feta, 1 oz (30 g)
Mozzarella, 1 oz (30 g)
Parmesan, 1 oz (30 g)
Port Salut, 1 oz (30 g)
Roquefort, 1 oz (30 g)
Swiss, 1 oz (30 g)

Milk Products

Lactose-free milk, low-fat or fat-free,
   8 fl oz (240 ml)
Milk, 1% or fat-free, 8 fl oz (240 ml)
Milk, whole, 8 fl oz (240 ml) – PLUS 2 Fat boxes
Skimmed dry milk, 5 tablespoons
Soya milk, fortified, 1% or fat-free, 8 fl oz (240 ml)
Yoghurt, frozen, low-fat or fat-free, 2 scoops
Yoghurt, low-fat or fat-free, flavoured, 8 oz (230 g)
   – PLUS 1 Fruit box and 2 Treats and Cravings
   boxes
Yoghurt, low-fat or fat-free, plain, 8 oz (230 g)
Yoghurt, whole milk, plain, 8 oz (230 g) – PLUS
   2 Fat boxes

protein

Unless otherwise specified, cross off 1 Protein box on your Eating Card for each specified amount. Higher-fat selections will require you to cross off 1 or 2 Fat boxes in addition to the Protein box. Meat protein sources are based on cooked portions; raw meat will shrink when cooking. A 4-oz (115-g) raw chicken breast will shrink to 3 oz (90 g) when cooked.

Preferred Proteins

Beans

Black, cooked, 3 oz (90 g)

Chickpeas, cooked, 3 oz (90 g)

Hummus, 4 level tablespoons – PLUS 1 Fat box

Kidney, cooked, 3 oz (90 g)

Lentils, cooked, 3 oz (90 g)

Lima, cooked, 3 oz (90 g)

Pinto, cooked, 3 oz (90 g)

Refried, fat-added, 3 oz (90 g) – PLUS 1 Fat box

Split peas, cooked, 3 oz (90 g)

White, cooked, 3 oz (90 g)

Eggs

Egg, whole, 1

Egg substitute, 4 tablespoons

Egg whites, 3

Poultry

Chicken or turkey, white meat without skin,
    1 oz (30 g)

Chicken or turkey, dark meat with skin,
    1 oz (30 g) – PLUS 1 Fat box

Seafood

Fish, canned

Salmon, packed in water, 2 oz (60 g)

Sardines, packed in water, 2 medium

Tuna, packed in water, 2 oz (60 g)

Fish, fresh or frozen

Flounder, 1 oz (30 g)

Fried fish, 1 oz (30 g) – PLUS 1 Fat box

Mahi mahi, 1 oz (30 g)

Salmon, 1 oz (30 g)

Sea bass, 1 oz (30 g)

Sole, 1 oz, (30 g)

Swordfish, 1 oz (30 g)

Tuna, 1 oz (30 g)

Shellfish

Clams, 2 oz (60 g)

Crab, 2 oz (60 g)

Crawfish, 2 oz (60 g)

Lobster, 2 oz (60 g)

Oysters, 6 medium

Prawns, 2 oz (60 g)

Scallops, 2 oz (60 g)

Soya Products

Soya beans, cooked, 3 oz (90 g)

Soya burger, ½ burger

Soya cheese, 1 oz (30 g)

Soya hot dog, 1

Soya milk, fortified, 1% or fat-
  free, 8 fl oz (240 ml)

Texturized soya protein, 1
  teaspoon or 1 oz (30 g)

Tofu, 3 oz (90 g)

Proteins to Minimize

Red Meats

Bacon, 1 rasher – PLUS 1 Fat
  box

Fillet steak, 1 oz (30 g)

Ham, smoked or fresh,
  1 oz (30 g)

Hot dog, beef or pork, 1 – PLUS
  2 Fat boxes

Lamb shank or shoulder, 1 oz
  (30 g)

Sirloin steak, 1 oz (30 g)

Stewing steak, 1 oz (30 g)

Topside, 1 oz (30 g)

Veal chop or roast, 1 oz (30 g)

Venison, 1 oz (30 g)

complex carbohydrates

Unless otherwise specified, cross off 1 Complex Carbohydrate box on your Eating Card for each specified amount. Higher-fat selections will require you to cross off 1 or 2 Fat boxes in addition to the Complex Carbohydrate box. If you can't find a particular complex carbohydrate listed, cross off one box for every 3 oz (90g) serving of cereal, grain, pasta or starchy vegetable. Remember that wholegrain products are ideal, but if you eat out or are travelling and whole grain products are not available, non-wholegrain versions are acceptable in moderation.

Preferred Carbohydrates

Wholegrain Breads

Bagel, ½ of a 2-oz (60-g) bagel

Bread, 1 oz (30 g) or 1 slice

English muffin, ½

Hamburger bun, ½

Naan bread, ¼ of 8 x 2 in (20 x 5 cm) loaf

Pitta bread 6-in (15-cm), ½

Roll, 1 small

Tortilla, corn, 6-in (15-cm), 1

Tortilla, flour, 7-inch (18-cm), 1

Waffle, fat-free, 1

Wholegrain Cereals and Grains

Barley, cooked, 3 oz (90 g)

Basmati rice, cooked, 2 oz (60 g)

Brown rice, cooked, 2 oz (60 g)

Buckwheat (kasha), cooked, 3 oz (90 g)

Bulgar wheat, cooked, 3 oz (90 g)

Cereal, cold, sweetened, ¾ oz (20 g)

Cereal, cold, unsweetened, 1 oz (30 g)

Cereal, hot, 3 oz (90 g)

Couscous, cooked, 3 oz (90 g)

Granola, low-fat, 1½ oz (45 g)

Jasmine rice, cooked, 2 oz (60 g)

Wheatgerm, 3 tablespoons

Wild rice, cooked, 2 oz (60 g)

Wholegrain Flour

Cornstarch, 2 tablespoons

Matzo meal, 5 tablespoons

Wholemeal flour, 2½ tablespoons

Wholegrain Pasta

Spelt and millet noodles, cooked spaghetti, 2½ oz (75 g)

Wholewheat spaghetti, cooked, 2½ oz (75 g)

Carbohydrates to Minimize

Starchy Vegetables
Butternut squash, 6½ oz (185 g)
Corn, 2½ oz (75 g)
Corn on the cob, 6-in (15-cm) ear
French fries, 10 – PLUS 1 Fat box
Green peas, 2½ oz (75 g)
Potato, baked, 1 small
Potato, instant, 2½ oz (75 g)
Potato, mashed, 4 oz (115 g)
Pumpkin, 4½ oz (125 g)
Sweet potato, 4 oz (115 g)

Crackers
Matzo, ¾ oz (20 g)
Melba toast, 4 slices
Wholewheat crackers, 2–5

vegetables

There are two kinds of vegetables in this section: limited ones, which are higher in calories, and unlimited ones. You may have as many of the unlimited vegetables as you wish. You don't have to cross off any Veggie boxes on your Eating Card for the unlimited ones. Vegetables that are high in starch do not appear on this list; they are on the Complex Carbohydrates list.

For each specified 'Limited Vegetable' amount, cross off 1 Veggie box on your Eating Card. All servings are 4 oz (115 g) raw or 2½ oz (75 g) cooked, unless otherwise specified.

Limited Vegetables

Artichoke, ½ medium

Aubergine

Asparagus

Bean sprouts

Beetroot

Broccoli

Brussels sprouts

Carrots

Cauliflower

Gherkins, 1½ large

Green beans

Green tomato, raw, 1 medium

Kale

Leeks

Mangetout

Onions

Parsnips

Peppers

Sauerkraut

Seaweed, raw

Snow peas

Swede

Tomato, 1 medium

Tomato paste, 3 tablespoons

Tomato purée, 4 fl oz (120 ml)

Tomatoes, canned, 4 oz (115 g)

Turnips

Vegetable soup, fat-free, low-sodium,
    4 fl oz (120 ml)

Unlimited Vegetables

Alfalfa sprouts

Cabbage

Celery

Chilli peppers

Courgettes

Cucumber

Garlic

Lettuce, all types

Mushrooms

Radishes

Spinach

Spring onions

Watercress

fruit

Unless otherwise specified, cross off 1 Fruit box on your Eating Card for each specified amount. If you can't find a particular fruit listed, cross off 1 box for every small to medium fresh fruit, 4½ oz (125 g) canned fruit, or 1½ oz (45 g) dried fruit.

Limited Fruit

Apple, green or red, 1 medium

Apple juice, 4 fl oz (120 ml)

Apple purée, unsweetened, 4 fl oz (120 ml)

Apricots, 4

Banana, ½ medium

Blackberries, 3½ oz (100 g)

Blueberries, 3½ oz (100 g)

Cantaloupe, ⅓ melon

Cherries, 12 large

Cranberry juice, 4 fl oz (120 ml)

Fruit salad, 4½ oz (125 g)

Grapefruit, ½

Grapefruit juice, 4 fl oz (120 ml)

Grapes, green or red, 12

Honeydew, ⅓ melon

Kiwifruit, 1 large

Orange, 1 medium

Orange juice, 4 fl oz (120 ml)

Peach, 1 medium

Pear, green, 1 small

Pineapple, canned, packed in juice, 4½ oz (125 g)

Plums, 2 medium

Prunes, 2

Raisins, 2 tablespoons

Raspberries, 4½ oz (125 g)

Strawberries, 4½ oz (125 g)

Watermelon, 1 cup cubed

Unlimited Fruit

Lemons

Limes

treats and cravings

Cross off 1 Treats and Cravings box on your Eating Card for each specified amount.

Biscuit with cream filling, 2 small – PLUS 1 Fat box

Biscuit, digestive, 1 small

Biscuits, fat-free, 2 small

Boiled sweets, 1

Brownie, 2 in (5 cm) square – PLUS 1 Fat box

Cake with icing, 1 in (2.5 cm) square – PLUS 1 Fat box

Cereal bar, 1 – PLUS 1 Fat box

Chicken rice soup, prepared with water, 4 fl oz (120 ml)

Chocolate candies (e.g. M&Ms), 6 pieces or 1 oz (30 g) – PLUS 1 Treats and Cravings box and 2 Fat boxes

Cocoa powder, 1 tablespoon

Cranberry sauce, 4 level tablespoons

Doughnut, ½ – PLUS 1 Fat box

Fortune cookie, 1

Fruit juice frozen bar, 1

Ice cream, 2½ oz (75 g) – PLUS 2 Fat boxes

Ice cream, light, 2½ oz (75 g) – PLUS 1 Fat box

Jelly, 4 oz (115 g)

Jelly beans, 7

Licorice twist, 1

Marshmallow, 1 large

Milk chocolate bar, 1.6 oz (50 g) – PLUS 1 Complex Carbohydrate box and 3 Fat boxes

Oatmeal biscuit, 1 medium – PLUS 1 Complex Carbohydrate box and 1 Fat box

Popcorn, fat-free, 2 handfuls

Potato crisps, fat-free, 15 to 20

Pretzels, unsalted, 10 small sticks

Rice cakes, mini, 2

Sorbet, 2 oz (60 g)

Table sugar, 1 teaspoon – PLUS 1 Complex Carbohydrate box

Tea, herbal, with 1 teaspoon honey, 1 cup

Tortilla chips, 6 to 12 – PLUS 2 Fat boxes

Tortilla chips, fat-free, 15 to 20

Vanilla wafers, 5 – PLUS 1 Fat box

Whipped topping, non-dairy, fat-free, 3 tablespoons

Wine gums, 8 small

alcohol

Cross off 2 Fat boxes for each of the specified amounts.

Beer – ½ pint (350 ml), PLUS 1 Complex
  Carbohydrate box

Spirits, 1½ fl oz (30 ml), roughly one standard
  measure
Wine, 5 fl oz (150 ml)

bonus items

Don't cross off any boxes.

Carbonated or sparkling water
  (add lime or lemon for great taste!)
Condiments: mustard, ketchup, barbecue sauce,
  brown sauce, fat-free salad dressing
  (3 tablespoons per day)
Diet drinks with aspartame and saccharin,
  2 per day

Green or herbal tea or decaffeinated coffee,
  2 cups per day
Non-stick cooking spray
Soda water
Tabasco sauce, hot-pepper sauce, pico de gallo,
  picante sauce

'Remember: eating a fat-free diet is the worst
thing you can do when you want to lose weight.'

fast foods

Busy, on-the-go lifestyles often means resorting to quick meals, whether it's a frozen dinner or takeaway. I recommend that you make your own meals, but here's a sampling of what to cross off on your Eating Cards for various meal combinations when you're short on time.

Chicken nuggets, 6: 1 Fat box; 2 Protein boxes; 1 Complex Carbohydrate box

Fish sandwich with tartar sauce, 1: 3 Fat boxes; 1 Protein box; 3 Complex Carbohydrate boxes

French fries, 20 to 25: 2 Fat boxes; 2 Complex Carbohydrate boxes

French stick sandwich, 6 in (15 cm): 1 Fat box; 2 Protein boxes; 3 Complex Carbohydrate boxes; 1 Veggie box

Fried chicken breast and wing, 1 each: 2 Fat boxes; 4 Protein boxes; 1 Complex Carbohydrate box

Hamburger, regular, 1: 2 Fat boxes; 2 Protein boxes; 2 Complex Carbohydrate boxes

Hot dog with bun, 1: 1 Fat box; 1 Protein box; 1 Complex Carbohydrate box

Pizza, thin crust with cheese, 3 small slices: 1 Fat box; 2 Protein boxes; 2 Complex Carbohydrate boxes

Pizza with meat topping, 3 small slices: 2 Fat boxes; 2 Protein boxes; 2 Complex Carbohydrate boxes

Taco, hard shell, 6 oz (170 g): 2 Fat boxes; 2 Protein boxes; 2 Complex Carbohydrate boxes

Taco, soft shell, 3 oz (90 g): 1 Fat box; 1 Protein box; 1 Complex Carbohydrate box

Turkey with gravy, mashed potatoes and dressing frozen dinner, 11 oz (300 g): 2 Fat boxes; 2 Protein boxes; 2 Complex Carbohydrate boxes

a week of eating...

The following menu contains exactly the number of calories and the breakdown of foods that you should eat during your *first week* of your 8 Minutes in the Morning programme.

I strongly urge you use this 'quick-start' menu as a guide for week 1. For weeks 2, 3, 4 and beyond, you will need to eat the appropriate number of calories on the Eating Card System (see page 75). You can move some food portions to other meals if you like; the only hard rule is that you can't move your fat. You must have fat with each main meal. You can also repeat or 'mix and match' the breakfasts, lunches or dinners as desired.

Day 1

breakfast
3 scrambled egg whites, 1 slice toast with 1 teaspoon flax or olive oil, 8 fl oz (240 ml) soya milk, ½ grapefruit, 1 cup green tea or decaffeinated coffee
1 protein, 1 complex carb, 1 fat, 1 dairy, 1 fruit

lunch
1 soya hot dog or 1 oz (30 g) sliced turkey on a bun with mustard and/or ketchup, 2½ oz (75 g) sweetcorn, large mixed green salad with 1 teaspoon flax oil, 3 oz (90 g) frozen low-fat yoghurt, 1 licorice twist
1 protein, 2 complex carbs, 2 veggies, 1 fat, 1 dairy, 1 treat/craving

dinner
½ BLT sandwich with avocado (1 slice bread with 1 oz (30 g) turkey bacon, iceberg lettuce, tomato, and ⅛ avocado), 8 fl oz (240 ml) tomato soup, 1 diet fizzy drink
1 complex carb, 1 protein, 2 veggies, 1 fat

snack
2 handfuls air-popped popcorn
1 treat/craving

...to get fit

Day 2

breakfast

1 oz (30 g) wholegrain cereal with 8 fl oz (240 ml) soya milk, 1 hard-boiled egg, 1 teaspoon flax oil, 1 small banana or ½ medium banana, 1 cup green tea or decaffeinated coffee

1 complex carb, 1 dairy, 1 protein, 1 fat, 1 fruit

lunch

8 fl oz (240 ml) lentil soup with 1 teaspoon flax oil added, medium wholegrain roll, large plate of steamed vegetables, 3 oz (90 g) frozen low-fat yoghurt, 1 fortune cookie, 1 glass soda water

1 protein, 1 fat, 1 complex carb, 2 veggies, 1 dairy, 1 treat/craving

dinner

Tuna pasta salad (2 oz (60 g), white tuna (water-packed) mixed with 1 tablespoon reduced-calorie mayonnaise, 2 tablespoons chopped onion and pickle, and 2½ oz (75 g) cooked penne pasta over lettuce), 1 small 6 in (15 cm), corn-on-the-cob, large plate of steamed vegetables, 1 sparkling water with lemon

1 protein, 1 fat, 2 complex carbs, 2 veggies

snack

2 mini rice cakes

1 treat/craving

Day 3

breakfast

½ toasted English muffin with 1 teaspoon flax oil, 3-egg-white omelette with vegetables, 1 glass soya milk, 1 apple, 1 cup green tea or decaffeinated coffee

1 complex carb, 1 fat, 1 protein, 1 veggie, 1 dairy, 1 fruit

lunch

½ turkey sandwich (1 slice bread with 1 oz (30 g) white-meat turkey, lettuce, tomato and mustard), 8 fl oz (240 ml) vegetable soup with 1 teaspoon flax oil added, 3 oz (90 g) frozen low-fat yoghurt, 1 diet fizzy drink

1 complex carb, 1 protein, 2 veggies, 1 fat, 1 dairy

dinner

Lettuce wrap (1 oz (30 g), white-meat chicken, 3 oz (90 g) brown rice and salsa wrapped in a large iceberg lettuce leaf large), large mixed green salad with 1 teaspoon of flax oil, 4 wholewheat crackers, 1 large marshmallow, 1 glass sparkling water with lemon

1 protein, 2 complex carbs, 1 veggie, 1 fat, 1 treat/craving

snack

2 fat-free biscuits

1 treat/craving

Day 4

breakfast
1½ oz (45 g) low-fat granola mixed with
4 oz (115 g) yoghurt and 4½ oz (125 g) fresh fruit
salad, 3 egg whites scrambled with 1 teaspoon flax oil,
1 cup green tea or decaffeinated coffee
1 complex carb, 1 dairy, 1 fruit, 1 protein, 1 fat

lunch
Chicken baked potato (1 small baked potato topped
with 1 oz (30 g) cubed sautéed chicken breast, 1 oz
(30 g) cheese and salsa), large plate of steamed
vegetables with 1 teaspoon flax oil, 4 oz (115 g) jelly,
1 glass soda water
**1 complex carb, 1 protein, 1 dairy, 2 veggies, 1 fat,
1 treat/craving**

dinner
Pasta with meat sauce (2½ oz (75 g) cooked pasta with
1 oz (30 g) cooked ground turkey breast, tomato sauce
and garlic), large mixed green salad with 1 teaspoon
flax oil, 1 bread roll, 1 diet fizzy drink
2 complex carbs, 1 protein, 2 veggies, 1 fat

snack
2 handfuls air-popped popcorn
1 treat/craving

Day 5

breakfast
Porridge made with with 1 oz (30 g) oats and 8 fl oz
(240 ml) soya milk, with 1 teaspoon flax oil added,
1 hard-boiled egg, ½ small bagel, 1 cup green tea or
decaffeinated coffee
2 complex carbs, 1 dairy, 1 fat, 1 protein

lunch
8 oz (230 g) chilli with 1 teaspoon flax oil added,
1 wholegrain tortilla, large plate of steamed vegetables,
3 oz (90 g) low-fat frozen yoghurt, 1 licorice twist,
1 glass sparkling water with lemon
**1 protein, 1 fat, 1 complex carb, 2 veggies, 1 dairy,
1 treat/craving**

dinner
Fajitas (1 oz (30 g) cooked chicken breast or beef,
3 oz (90 g) onions and peppers sautéed with cooking
oil spray, then wrapped in a tortilla with tomato, lettuce
and 2 tablespoons guacamole), 4½ oz (125 g) fruit
salad, 1 diet fizzy drink
1 protein, 2 veggies, 1 complex carb, 1 fat, 1 fruit

snack
1 small digestive biscuit
1 treat/craving

Day 6

breakfast
1 slice toast with 2 teaspoons peanut or almond butter, 1 oz (30 g) cooked ham, 2 oz (60 g) plain low-fat yoghurt mixed with 4½ oz (125 g) strawberries, 1 cup green tea or decaffeinated coffee
1 complex carb, 1 fat, 1 protein, 1 dairy, 1 fruit

lunch
Tuna pitta (2 oz (60 g) white tuna (water-packed) mixed with 1 tablespoon low-calorie mayonnaise spooned into ½ pitta with lettuce and tomato), 8 fl oz (240 g) vegetable soup, 3 oz (90 g) frozen low-fat yoghurt, 2 tablespoons raisins, 1 diet fizzy drink
1 protein, 1 fat, 1 complex carb, 2 veggies, 1 dairy, 1 treat/craving

dinner
1 oz (30 g) grilled salmon with grilled onions and garlic, 2 oz (60 g) rice, large green salad with 1 tablespoon oil-based dressing, 8 small wine gums, 1 glass soda water
1 protein, 1 complex carb, 2 veggies, 1 fat, 1 treat/craving

snack
½ small bagel
1 complex carb

Day 7

breakfast
Breakfast burrito (1 small wholewheat tortilla filled with 3 scrambled egg whites, 1 oz (30 g) cheese, 1 teaspoon flax oil, and salsa), 1 apple, 1 cup green tea or decaffeinated coffee
1 complex carb, 1 protein, 1 dairy, 1 fat, 1 fruit

lunch
Turkey melt (1 slice wholewheat toast topped with 1 oz (30 g) white-meat turkey and 1 slice soya or regular cheese, then grilled for 2 minutes), large mixed green salad with 1 teaspoon flax oil, 1 licorice twist, 1 diet fizzy drink
1 complex carb, 1 protein, 1 dairy, 1 veggie, 1 fat, 1 treat/craving

dinner
Chinese stir-fry (1 oz (30 g) chicken breast or beef, 2 cups vegetables stir-fried with water, pepper, and low-sodium soy sauce over 1 oz (30 g) brown rice), large mixed green salad with 1 teaspoon flax oil, 1 bread roll, 1 glass sparkling water with lemon
1 protein, 3 veggies, 2 complex carbs, 1 fat

snack
2 handfuls air-popped popcorn
1 treat/craving

jorge's recipes

Here are some great healthy recipes, most chock-full of veggies, to help keep you going strong in weeks 2, 3, 4 and beyond of the Eat Fat to Get Fit programme.

chinese veggie stir-fry

1 protein box, 2 veggie boxes

4 fl oz (120 ml) soy sauce,
 low-sodium if possible
4 fl oz (120 ml) water
3 oz (90 g) tofu, cubed (optional)
3 oz (90 g) chopped white onion
4 cloves garlic, crushed
4 oz (115 g) broccoli florets
1 tablespoon fresh ginger, finely
chopped2 small carrots, sliced
8 oz (230 g) mushrooms, sliced
½ cup snow pea pods
½ cup diced celery
¼ cup sliced water chestnuts

In a wok or large frying pan, heat the soy sauce and water over high heat. Add the tofu (if using), onion and garlic. Sauté for 2 minutes. Add the broccoli, ginger and carrots. Sauté for 4 minutes. Add the mushrooms, pea pods, celery and water chestnuts. Continue to stir-fry until the vegetables are *al dente*. You may add more water or soy sauce, if desired. *Makes 6 servings*

chinese broccoli and cauliflower salad
1 veggie box, 1½ fat boxes

1 lb (455 g) broccoli florets

1 lb (455 g) cauliflower florets

1 tablespoon olive oil

2 tablespoons sesame oil

4 tablespoons soy sauce, low-sodium if possible

6 spring onions, chopped

4 cloves garlic, crushed

In a large saucepan, blanch the broccoli and cauliflower in plenty of boiling water for 3 minutes. Drain in a colander and rinse with cold water. Combine the olive oil, sesame oil, soy sauce, spring onions and garlic in a medium bowl. Mix in the broccoli and cauliflower. Chill before serving. *Makes 6 servings*

cucumber-tomato salad
1 veggie box

4 plum tomatoes, chopped

3 cucumbers, peeled, seeded and chopped

1 tablespoon olive oil

Salt and pepper, to taste

In a medium bowl, mix the tomatoes, cucumbers and oil. Season with the salt and pepper. Chill before serving. *Makes 6 servings*

grilled chicken salad
2 protein boxes, 3 veggie boxes, 1 fat box

2 oz (60 g) grilled chicken breast

2 handfuls lettuce

2 tomatoes, diced

2 small carrots, grated

1 tablespoon dressing

In a large bowl, toss together the chicken, lettuce, tomato and carrot. Add the dressing and mix well. *Makes 1 serving*

pasta with veggies
2 complex carbohydrate boxes, 2 veggie boxes, 1 fat box

1 tablespoon olive oil

2 tomatoes, chopped

1 courgette, sliced

4 oz (115 g) mushrooms, sliced

1 large handful of fresh basil leaves, torn

2 cloves garlic, crushed

Freshly ground black pepper, to taste

4 oz (115 g) cooked wholewheat pasta

Heat the oil in a large frying pan. Sauté the tomato, courgettes, mushrooms, basil and garlic over medium-high heat until tender. Season with the pepper. Serve the pasta topped with the vegetables. *Makes 1 serving*

egg-white scramble
1 protein box, 1 veggie box

1 tomato, chopped
½ small onion, chopped
4 mushrooms, chopped
½ courgette, chopped
3 egg whites
4 tablespoons salsa

Coat a medium frying pan with cooking oil spray. Scramble the tomato, onion, mushrooms and courgette into the egg whites. Top with the salsa. *Makes 1 serving*

three-bean salad
1 protein box, 2 veggie boxes, 1 fat box

2 oz (60 g) cooked chickpeas
2 oz (60 g) cooked kidney beans
3 oz (90 g) steamed green beans
½ small red onion, chopped
1 teaspoon olive oil
1 tomato, diced
1 teaspoon balsamic vinegar
2 handfuls salad leaves

In a medium bowl, toss the chickpeas, kidney beans and green beans with the onion, oil, tomato and vinegar. Serve on a bed of salad leaves. *Makes 1 serving*
Variation: Use canned mixed beans.

roasted chicken

2 protein boxes

2 oz (60 g) skinless, boneless chicken breast

1 tablespoon fresh sage, chopped

1 tablespoon fresh rosemary, chopped

Preheat the oven to 180°C/350°F/gas mark 4. Coat the chicken with cooking oil spray. Sprinkle evenly with the sage and rosemary. Roast for 45 minutes or until a meat thermometer inserted in the thickest portion registers 70°C/160°F and the juices run clear. *Makes 1 serving*

burrito

1 complex carbohydrate box, 2 protein boxes, 1 veggie box, 1 fat box

3 oz (90 g) refried beans

1 handful lettuce, shredded

1 oz (30 g) soya cheese, grated

1 wholewheat tortilla, 7-inch (18-cm)

4 tablespoons salsa

Wrap the refried beans, lettuce and cheese in the tortilla. Place the tortilla in a small cast-iron frying pan and heat over medium heat until both sides are slightly brown. Remove and top with the salsa. *Makes 1 serving*

pitta pizza
2 complex carbohydrate boxes, 1 protein box, 1 veggie box, 1 fat box

1 teaspoon olive oil

4 oz (115 g) broccoli, chopped and steamed

2 tomatoes, chopped

1 large handful fresh basil, torn

1 clove garlic, crushed

1 wholewheat pitta bread

1 oz (30 g) mozzarella-style soya cheese

Heat the oil in a frying pan. Sauté the broccoli, tomato, basil and garlic over medium-high heat. Spoon the mixture into the pitta and sprinkle with cheese. Grill for 1 to 2 minutes, until the cheese melts.
Makes 1 serving

tuna melt
1 complex carbohydrate box, 2 protein boxes, 1 fat box

2 oz (60 g) water-packed tuna

1 tablespoon red onion, chopped

1 tablespoon gherkin, chopped

1 tablespoon reduced-calorie or soya mayonnaise

1 slice wholewheat bread

1 oz (30 g) Cheddar-style soya cheese

Preheat the grill. Mix the tuna with the onion, gherkin and mayonnaise. Spoon the mixture onto the bread and top with the cheese. Grill for 1 to 2 minutes, or until the cheese melts. *Makes 1 serving*

hot veggie pitta sandwich
2 complex carbohydrate boxes, 1 protein box, 3 veggie boxes

12 oz (340 g) vegetables, chopped

½ small onion, chopped

1 clove garlic, crushed

1 wholewheat pitta bread

1 oz (30 g) soya cheese, grated

Coat a large frying pan with cooking oil spray. Sauté the vegetables, onion and garlic over medium-high heat. Slice the pitta in half and stuff each half with the mixture. Add the cheese. *Makes 1 serving*

salmon salad
1 protein box, 2 veggie boxes, 1 fat box

2 oz (60 g) grilled or canned salmon

½ small red onion, chopped

1 tomato, chopped

1 carrot, grated

6 mushrooms, sliced

2 handfuls lettuce, shredded

1 tablespoon reduced-calorie dressing

In a medium bowl, toss the salmon, onion, tomato, carrot and mushrooms with the lettuce. Add the dressing and mix well. *Makes 1 serving*

chicken fajitas
**2 complex carbohydrate boxes, 1 protein box,
1½ veggie boxes**

2 oz (60 g) chicken breast, sliced

1 onion, sliced

1 red pepper, sliced

1 green pepper, sliced

Freshly ground black pepper, to taste

2 wholewheat or corn tortillas, 7-inch (18-cm)

Coat a medium frying pan with cooking oil spray. Sauté the chicken, onion and red and green peppers over medium-high heat. Season with the black pepper. Spoon the mixture into the tortillas and roll up to enclose the filling. *Makes 2 servings*

the eat fat to get fit
eating card system

Eating the best kinds of food in the right amounts is key to being successful in your weight-loss journey. I have created Eating Cards to take all the guesswork out of it for you.

First, draw a thick line over the dotted line next to your calorie selection (see page 75). In the sample card, the line is to the right of the Quick Start. The boxes to the left are the servings of each food you can enjoy each day. Mark off the boxes corresponding to the type and amount of food you eat. Here, the person has eaten the recommended breakfast and lunch from the Quick Start menu (on page 226) plus 5 glasses of water. The uncrossed boxes show what she can eat for dinner and any snacks. When all the boxes are crossed off, you have finished eating for the rest of the day.

I've included two master Eating Cards opposite.

Photocopy them and keep them with you all the time. It's easier to mark them as the day goes on, so you don't forget. Just cut the cards on the dotted lines, stack them, and staple them in the upper left-hand corner to make a little booklet. You can put the booklet into an old chequebook cover to protect it and make it very convenient to use!

Your Eating Card System

Draw a thick line over the dotted line to the right of your calorie selection. Everything to the left is your daily food intake.

Date: _____

	Quick Start (Week 1) ◄	1,200 ◄	1,400 ◄	1,600 ◄	1,800 ◄	2,000 ◄
Fats	☒ ☒ ☐	☐		☐	☐ ☐	☐
Proteins	☒ ☒ ☐	☐	☐	☐		☐
Complex Carbs	☒ ☒ ☒ ☐			☐	☐	☐
Dairy	☒ ☒					
Veggies	☒ ☒ ☐ ☐	☐	☐			
Fruits	☒					
Treats/Cravings	☒ ☐				☐	
Water	☒ ☒ ☒ ☒ ☒ ☐ ☐ ☐					

www.jorgecruise.com

Instructions for blank Eating Cards: Make four copies for each week. Cut on the dotted lines, then stack and staple in the upper left-hand corner. Keep them with you at all times.

Your Eating Card System

Draw a thick line over the dotted line to the right of your calorie selection. Everything to the left is your daily food intake.

Date: _____

	Quick Start (Week 1) ◄	1,200 ◄	1,400 ◄	1,600 ◄	1,800 ◄	2,000 ◄
Fats	☐ ☐ ☐	☐		☐	☐ ☐	☐
Proteins	☐ ☐ ☐	☐	☐	☐		☐
Complex Carbs	☐ ☐ ☐ ☐		☐	☐	☐	☐
Dairy	☐ ☐					
Veggies	☐ ☐ ☐ ☐	☐	☐			
Fruits	☐					
Treats/Cravings	☐ ☐				☐	
Water	☐ ☐ ☐ ☐ ☐ ☐ ☐ ☐	www.jorgecruise.com				

Your Eating Card System

Draw a thick line over the dotted line to the right of your calorie selection. Everything to the left is your daily food intake.

Date: _____

	Quick Start (Week 1) ◄	1,200 ◄	1,400 ◄	1,600 ◄	1,800 ◄	2,000 ◄
Fats	☐ ☐ ☐	☐		☐	☐ ☐	☐
Proteins	☐ ☐ ☐	☐	☐	☐		☐
Complex Carbs	☐ ☐ ☐ ☐		☐	☐	☐	☐
Dairy	☐ ☐					
Veggies	☐ ☐ ☐ ☐	☐	☐			
Fruits	☐					
Treats/Cravings	☐ ☐				☐	
Water	☐ ☐ ☐ ☐ ☐ ☐ ☐ ☐	www.jorgecruise.com				

become a weight-loss star

Here's a motivational incentive to keep you going. Send me your weight-loss success story and you will qualify to have your story appear on my website. You will also be put in the running to qualify to meet me in person in San Diego, California! Plus, if you are selected, I might feature you during my television appearances, in my magazine columns, on my website or in forthcoming books. You'll become a weight-loss star! It will not only acknowledge your hard work but also help inspire others to improve their lives. Get ready to step up and become part of my weight-loss revolution!

here's how it works

Each year, I host a red rose ceremony in San Diego for my most inspirational and successful clients. With help from my staff, I pick 20 people for the yearly trip.

You will receive a free makeover, new wardrobe and a VIP maintenance plan, designed exclusively for you (a value of over £6,000). At the ceremony, I will recognize you in front of an auditorium filled with more than 200 people and capture the event on camera. So, are you ready to become an inspirational role model to millions?

To apply, visit *www.jorgecruise.com/redrose* and download your Red Rose Success Story form. Fill it out and mail it, along with your 'before' and 'after' photos, to the address listed on the form.

about the author

Jorge (pronounced HOR-hay) Cruise is the New York Times bestselling author of the *8 Minutes in the Morning*® book series and is recognized as the number one online weight-loss specialist, due to his unprecedented success in helping more than 3 million people lose weight at his web site *www.jorgecruise.com*. No other weight-loss specialist has had so many people directly reveal what really works to make them consistently losing 2 pounds each week in just 8 minutes. This makes Jorge one of the most up-to-date and in-demand weight loss specialists both online and offline.

Jorge has been featured in the *New York Times*, *USA Today*, *People Magazine*, *Woman's World*, *First for Women*, *Self*, *Shape*, *Cosmo*, *Fit* and has appeared on Oprah, CNN, Good Morning America, Dateline NBC, Extra and Lifetime.

Jorge is also a nominee for Fitness Instructor of the Year by IDEA – a national association of fitness professionals – and was named by Arnold Schwarzenegger as a special advisor to the California Governor's Council on Physical Fitness and Sports.

In addition, 11 million people read his monthly column called the 'Weight Loss Coach' in *Prevention* magazine. Jorge is also a member of the Association of Health Care Journalists, a non-profit organization dedicated to advancing public understanding of health care issues. He is fluent in both English and Spanish.

Utilizing the knowledge and credentials that he has gained from the University of California, San Diego (UCSD), Dartmouth College, the Cooper Institute for Aerobics Research, the American College of Sports Medicine (ACSM) and the American Council on Exercise (ACE), Jorge is dedicated to helping time-deprived women, men, kids and seniors lose weight and achieve their dreams.

He lives in San Diego, California with his wife Heather. He can be contacted via *www.jorgecruise.com*.

photo credits

Front cover photo © Robert Trachtenberg
Back cover photos courtesy of Jorge Cruise
Interior photos by Mitch Mandel/Rodale Images, except the following:
Courtesy of Jorge Cruise: pp. 12, 15, 22, 23, 25, 26, 34, 51, 53, 54, 111, 112, 140, 168, 196, 201
Courtesy of Rodale Images: pp. 71, 73

index

d

S

y

OTHER RODALE BOOKS
AVAILABLE FROM PAN MACMILLAN

1-4050-0666-8	Banish Your Belly, Butt & Thighs Forever!	*The Editors of* Prevention *Health Books for Women*	£10.99
1-4050-0665-X	Get A Real Food Life	*Janine Whiteson*	£12.99
1-4050-0667-6	The Green Pharmacy	*Dr James A. Duke*	£14.99
1-4050-0673-0	The Home Workout Bible	*Lou Schuler*	£15.99
1-4050-0674-9	The Hormone Connection	*Maleskey and Kittel*	£15.99
1-4050-0671-4	Laying Down the Law	*Dr Ruth Peters*	£8.99
1-4050-0672-2	Pilates for Every Body	*Denise Austin*	£12.99
1-4050-0669-2	The Testosterone Advantage Plan™	*Lou Schuler*	£12.99
1-4050-0668-4	Whole Body Meditations	*Lorin Roche*	£10.99
1-4050-0670-6	Win the Fat War	*Anne Alexander*	£5.99

All Pan Macmillan titles can be ordered from our website, *www.panmacmillan.com,* or from your local bookshop and are also available by post from:

Bookpost, PO Box 29, Douglas, Isle of Man IM99 1BQ
Credit cards accepted. For details:
Telephone: 01624 836000
Fax: 01624 670923
E-mail: bookshop@enterprise.net
www.bookpost.co.uk

Free postage and packing in the United Kingdom

Prices shown above were correct at time of going to press.
Pan Macmillan reserve the right to show new retail prices on covers which may differ from those previously advertised in the text or elsewhere.

RODALE   MACMILLAN